The Wild Remedy

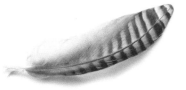

How Nature Mends Us

~ A Diary

EMMA MITCHELL

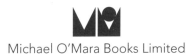

Michael O'Mara Books Limited

This paperback edition first published in 2021
First published in Great Britain in 2019 by
Michael O'Mara Books Limited
9 Lion Yard
Tremadoc Road
London SW4 7NQ

A CIP catalogue record for this book is available from the British Library.

Papers used by Michael O'Mara Books Limited are natural, recyclable
products made from wood grown in sustainable forests. The manufacturing
processes conform to the environmental regulations of the country of origin.

ISBN: 978-1- 78929-290-9 in paperback print format
ISBN: 978-1-78929-046-2 in ebook format

1 2 3 4 5 6 7 8 9 10

www.mombooks.com

Interior and cover photography and illustration by Emma Mitchell
Cover design by Claire Cater
Designed and typeset by Claire Cater

Printed and bound in China

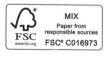

MIX
Paper from
responsible sources
FSC
www.fsc.org   FSC® C016973

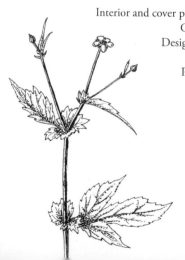

Contents

For Rachael

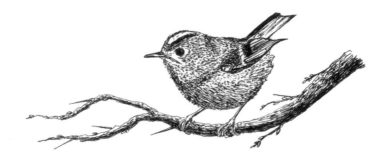

Introduction

I'm not going to mince my words: I suffer from depression and have done for twenty-five years. Some days my brain feels as though it is mired in a dark quicksand of negativity; on others, layers of thick greyish cloud seem to descend, weighing down my thoughts and burgling my motivation. However the depression manifests itself, I find it difficult to move, and the urge to stay nestled indoors beneath a quilt and near to Netflix is strong. I know that if I do force myself to get up from the sofa, then the gloom can lift a little, and if I step outside and walk in the wood behind our cottage, the dreich thoughts may not leave entirely but they certainly retreat to the wings. For me, taking a daily walk among plants and trees is as medicinal as any talking cure or pharmaceutical. I know this sounds like an advice leaflet from a Victorian sanatorium, and there are echoes of the bracing strictures of a previous age here, but only in the last year have I realized quite how beneficial being in a green place can be, even if it is only for five or ten minutes. Simply getting out of the house and seeing the blackthorns and lime tree opposite our cottage induces a response in me that I can only describe as a neuronal sigh of relief: an unseen, silent reaction in the brain that is simultaneously soothing and curative.

Of course, I am not the first to have noticed the consolation of walking outdoors. Literature is peppered with references to striding in the countryside as a means of easing melancholy, inspiring creative thought and hastening recovery. The nineteenth-century

Danish philosopher, poet and theologian, Søren Kierkegaard, exalted a daily stroll: 'Every day I walk myself into a state of well-being and walk away from every illness; I have walked myself into my best thoughts, and I know of no thought so burdensome that one cannot walk away from it.' Elizabeth von Arnim wrote one of my favourite novels, *The Enchanted April*, in the 1920s, and her feelings on walking through the countryside echo my own: 'If you go to a place on anything but your own feet you are taken there too fast, and miss a thousand delicate joys that were waiting for you by the wayside.'

When I walk the half-mile or so from our front door to the entrance of the village wood, follow the mown paths that trail between the trees and begin to notice the plants going to seed or coming into flower, seek out the yellow-striped grove snail shells part-hidden in the chalky soil and catch sight of a muntjac deer as it scampers away, the mental relief I felt at seeing that lime tree opposite our cottage is multiplied many-fold. I become engrossed in every leafy, creeping or flying inhabitant of the wood, and with each detail that draws my attention, with each metre I walk, the incessant clamour of daily concerns seems to become more muffled and the foggy pall of depression begins to disperse.

I remember squatting on my haunches as a small child near my paternal grandparents' house in North Wales, gazing at a tangle of bluebell buds, hawthorn leaves, spikes of ground ivy and seedlings of cleavers beneath a hedge, wondering at the patterns they made and the innumerable shades of green on display, and being enchanted. From an early age it was the sight of these small but complex botanical jumbles that first shifted my neurons into a mode of elated awe. I remember thinking that it felt as though a bubble was expanding in my mind. It helped to distract from difficult days, then as it does now. If a moth or a beetle entered the scene as I watched, intent upon some journey or task, then the feelings of wonder became more intense. A very small story was unfolding in front of me: I was seeing a snapshot of that creature's life and I felt thrilled and privileged to witness it. I will still squat, aged forty-six, to examine humble yet exquisite collections of plants or lichens growing on the pebbles of Dungeness or the small creatures that dart about in rock pools. The nineteenth-century poet John Clare called this 'dropping down', and he did it too, sitting among wild plants to see the natural world from the point of view of a snipe in its nest. This physical and mental immersal in nature informed and inspired his verse.

The sight of a path curving gently through hazels, a great stand of beeches, the sweep of the white sands and calm water of Shell Bay in Dorset, or the monumental yet softly cat-like Howgill Fells in Cumbria, is undeniably uplifting and beautiful. The promise of seeing a blue tit or a wild orchid may draw us outside, and innumerable passages in literature urge us to take to the countryside if we wish to send melancholy packing, but is there a scientific basis for the positive feelings that nature seems to confer? Might there be measurable changes in our brains and bodies when we walk the Downs or step into a bluebell wood in May? There are. Joint research from the University of Madrid and the Norwegian University of Life Sciences published in 2007, for instance, showed that simply seeing natural landscapes can speed up recovery from stress or mental fatigue, and hasten recovery from illness. Studies published in 2017 from the University of Exeter have demonstrated that the presence of vegetation in an urban landscape diminishes levels of depression, anxiety and perceived stress levels in city dwellers, and the same raft of work showed that time spent outdoors alleviates low mood.

More recently, popular attention has been caught by a concept from Japan and China called *Shinrin-yoku* or 'forest bathing'. It is a common practice that began in the early 1980s, involving spending time in a wood or forest to 'bathe' in the atmosphere for the benefit of mind and body. Around a quarter of the population of Japan have tried this therapy at forty-eight officially designated forest bathing trails, and when I first read about it I was thrilled. It is the process I have just described: it is what I do most days to alleviate my low mood, yet continents away in a different culture this process of botanically-based self-medication is used by millions of people to ease the symptoms of both physical and mental illness. It is no more unusual to seek out trees and plants when feeling unwell in Japan than it is to nip to the chemist for some ibuprofen in the UK.

In recent years, follow-up research aimed at understanding the *Shinrin-yoku* phenomenon has shown that walking in a green space has a direct positive effect on several systems in our bodies. Blood pressure decreases, levels of the stress hormone cortisol drop, anxiety is alleviated and pulse rates diminish in subjects who have spent time in nature and particularly among trees. Levels of activity in the sympathetic nervous system, responsible for our fight or flight response to stress, drop away, and the activity of a particular kind of white blood cell called natural killer (NK) cells, which can destroy virally infected and certain cancerous cells, increases when humans spend time in a woodland environment. These biochemical changes lasted for up to a month in the subjects who took part in these studies; the effects were not observed when they spent the same length of time in a city. The mental sigh of relief I feel when I see the trees opposite our cottage is not simply caused by my fondness for looking at bonny bosky views; I am experiencing real physiological responses that affect my body and mind.

What are the biochemical mechanisms by which wild places alleviate depression and improve health in humans?

Further research is beginning to provide tangible clues. Many plant species produce volatile compounds and oils, collectively known as phytoncides, in order to fight infection from viruses and bacteria. Studies from the academic groups that examined the *Shinrin-yoku* phenomenon have shown that inhalation of phytoncides triggers some of the same effects on our immune, endocrine (hormonal), circulatory and nervous systems. These oils do not have to be highly scented to have an effect on our bodies and most aren't. The fresh 'green' smell of a hedgerow in May is a combination of phytoncides from many different plants. We inhale them without realizing it when we spend time in a wild place.

We see further clues when we interrogate serotonin levels. Serotonin is a compound that carries signals between nerve cells in our brain, and the levels of this neurotransmitter are diminished in depressed patients. It is not yet clear whether this shift in serotonin is a cause of low mood or one of its effects, and there are certainly other mechanisms in the brain that are involved in the regulation of mood, but there does seem to be a link between serotonin and mood in humans, and interacting with the natural world has been shown to influence serotonin levels. Indeed, just being outside can make a difference: when sunlight hits the skin or the eye's retina it triggers the release of serotonin, and on brighter days higher levels are released. It is the lower levels of sunshine between November and March that leads to winter depression or Seasonal Affective Disorder (SAD) in some individuals. I am prone to this form of transient seasonal sadness and it can make the winter months especially challenging.

Another, more surprising, way in which interacting with the natural world influences our serotonin levels comes from the soil. When humans come into contact with benign soil bacteria such as *Mycobacterium vaccae*, proteins from its cell wall trigger a further release of serotonin from a specific group of nerve cells in our brains. So it seems that a bit of weeding can be good for more than just your herbaceous borders.

Finally, when we take some light exercise, such as walking, endorphins are released into the bloodstream. These are neurotransmitters that diminish the sensation of pain and induce a mild euphoria: a gentle, natural high. Combine these with the effects of light from the sun, compounds from the plants and benevolent bacteria from the soil, and it seems that walking in a garden, field or wood is like reaching into an invisible natural medicine cabinet. The science is still progressing, and there is clearly much more to discover, but I'm fascinated by the idea that the balance of the chemistry of my brain, and my hormonal and nervous systems, are changing as I linger among trees and plants and that this can impact the tone of my thoughts and my mental health. I have felt the curative effects of my surroundings as I walk in a wild place innumerable times, and it is reassuring to know that there is something I can do to help myself on dark days.

For me, it is the combination of experiencing the large-scale elements of a landscape, then casting my eyes down to examine the intricate minuscule world that exists on a tree stump or along a grass verge, that makes the biggest difference to my state of mind. When I am walking, my mind enters a state of very careful noticing. I seek out collections of plants, empty snail shells, berries and seed heads. As I do so I feel as though I'm swimming in the small details I see, so deeply do I become immersed in my surroundings. I feel strongly that this is an ancient foraging instinct; it distracts and seems to muffle worries and root my mind in the present as I walk. I use it as a sort of wild yoga, and my searching results in small seasonal collections of common plants, flowers and nature finds that I photograph and hoard.

The book that helps me to decode the medley of plants I see on my walks and put names to leaves and flowers is one I found in my grandad's bookcase in 1978. The dust-jacket drew me in: it was covered in a beautiful array of wild roses, their hips and leaves. I opened it at random and entered a botanical wonderland. Many of the plates in *The Concise British Flora in Colour* resemble the base of a hedgerow in March or a woodland floor in mid-June, and I was enthralled by them and still am. Its author, Reverend William Keble Martin (1877–1969), began painting watercolours of the wildflowers of Britain in his twenties and was eighty-eight when the book was published. He dedicated most of his life to creating this exquisite book and over 1,400 of his small paintings cover its plates. Individually, they are quietly beautiful, botanically accurate, and have helped thousands of people identify something they may have found in a field on their holidays or growing between paving stones up their road. Together, though, the collection of paintings on each plate is astonishingly beautiful.

It is the intricate, sometimes tangled arrangement of Keble Martin's paintings that draws me in and ensures that I keep returning to the book's pages. He composed each plate almost as though the plants are competing for light and finding their space in a jumbled patch on the edge of a cemetery or on a piece of waste ground. If you look skywards while standing in a wood you will notice that the branches of trees do not overlap. Their growth stops short, leaving a small gap between the branches of adjacent individuals, giving a tantalizing hint at the existence of inter-tree communication: a sort of agreement between neighbouring trees that enables them to maximize the harvesting of light in a limited space. Keble Martin's plates covered in collections of wildflower paintings present a sort of miniature version of this 'crown shyness'. The way the specimens are set out in this book speaks of hundreds of hours studying the manner in which wild plants grow in relation to one another.

Keble Martin's beautiful, naturalistic compositions mean that on days when my depressive thoughts are overwhelming, simply looking at the plates in *The Concise British Flora in Colour* can bring some of the relief I feel when I'm out in the countryside. I open it when depression has frozen my mind in a kind of mental winter, and it allows me to peep into spring without leaving the living room. This book is an antidepressant made of paper and ink.

The drive to be among, gaze at and in some cases bring home plants, insects, shells, birds and mammals and the things they leave behind is accompanied by a compulsion to record my sightings and finds in some way. Photography often answers this need, but I frequently feel the need to draw certain species that I become particularly familiar with. I wonder if this might be a version of our ancestors' urge to paint images on the walls of their shelters or caves of the animals they observed and hunted, such as those at Lascaux in France. Perhaps those paintings were intended to show the immense respect the painters felt for those animals and the awe they inspired; this is exactly why I take up pencil or pen after my walks. The cave paintings may also have been driven by gratitude felt towards some of those species for providing a source of food. I must emphasize that I do not eat any of the creatures I paint – no voles were barbecued in the making of this book – but if I see a robin I am exhilarated; that sighting can help to alleviate melancholy, and I am keen to paint the robin in order, perhaps, to hold on to that effect for a little longer.

In my first book, *Making Winter*, I wrote about the benefit to mental health of time spent in creative activity; I find that making a simple sketch of shepherd's purse, a watercolour of a goldcrest or gathering specimens to make a herbarium of common botanical finds is as soothing to my mind as the walk itself. Making a passable pencil likeness of a sparrowhawk can be as effective at diverting my mind from difficult, dark thoughts as the encounter with the bird that inspired it, and the gently repetitive process of looking and drawing is far more important than a perfect result. The beneficial effects of nature sightings and the time I spend recording what I have seen seem to be synergistic in some way. I could not write a book about a year of nature walks without including my drawings, paintings and photographs.

When I spend time in a wild place or a garden and notice the small details of the plants, trees and wildlife that inhabit it, the symptoms of my depression are eased, and this has become a way in which I self-medicate. At no point would I suggest that standard treatments for this condition be replaced by dawdling near a dog rose: I rely on antidepressants and talking cures to prevent my illness from becoming overwhelming, but depression varies in its grip on my mind, depending on the season and on daily stress levels. I have found that the basal level of respite provided by antidepressants and therapy is sometimes insufficient to prevent my thoughts falling down a well. It is at these times that I find walking among hazels and hawthorns can help to dial down cortisol levels and cause the shift in neurotransmitters that I need to fend off the black dog. Walking several times a week, even on days when I feel well, seems to have a cumulative effect and can help to make the dips in mood less vertiginous.

Going for a walk among trees or in a field is something you can do if life is generally all right, to help you to get through the usual doldrums and jaggedly stressful days that do and will arrive. When life is incessantly exhausting, has thrown you a terrible gluey lump of pain and you feel dreadfully, dingily sad, a leafy place and the sight of a bird in it can divert and begin to heal the mind. It's something you can do if you have a deadline that feels like doom, your to-do list is as long as the M4 or you are waiting for antidepressants to take effect. My hope is that if low mood has you pinned to your sofa or bed and you feel as though you are wading through the treacle of sadness, reading about what I have seen, seeing the photographs and illustrations in this book, and perhaps venturing out to seek a winkle or a weasel of your own, may bring some relief. Walk; walk or wheel yourself outside if you can; seek out green, where furred or feathered things might be, even in your back garden. It really will help.

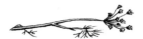

This is a book about what I see when I venture outside our cottage over the course of a year, both on days when the effort needed to do so seems too much to surmount and when all is well and the sunshine and birdsong call to me. None of the sightings I describe are terribly unusual: there are no close encounters with golden eagles and I don't make friends with a Scottish wildcat. Apart from a tiny orchid that I shinned up a hill to find, the species I write about in this book are relatively common and many can be seen in urban parks. I've written about how standing among a carpet of jewel-like autumn leaves, finding some newly emerged catkins, or spotting a sparrowhawk skimming across a stubble field, can bring solace. As the novelist Alice Walker wrote: 'I understood at a very early age that in nature, I felt everything I should feel in church but never did.'

If you would like to read in more depth about the research mentioned in this introduction, there is a list of further reading at the back of the book.

Pathway in Fermyn Woods, Northamptonshire >

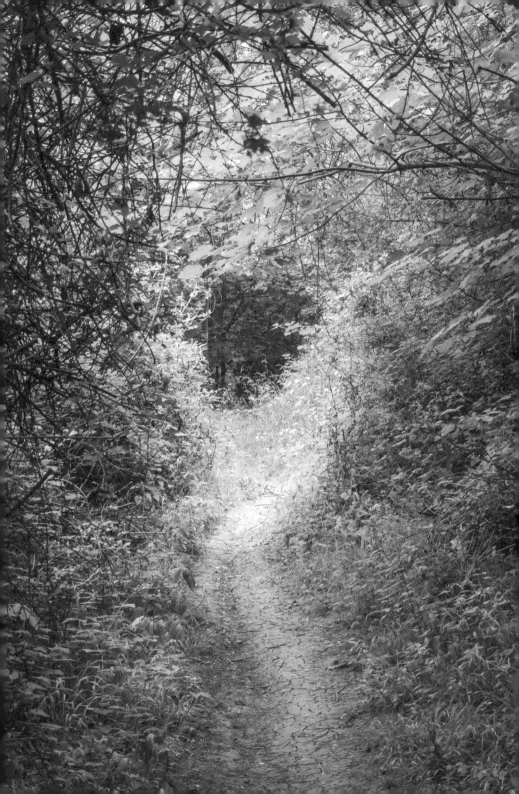

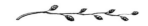

Flora & Fauna

(Key sightings)

KEY: colloquial names, collective noun

OCTOBER

Blue fleabane (*Erigeron acer*)
Cleavers (*Galium aparine*); bort, bedstraw,
  sticky weed, sticky bobs, sticky willy, sticky
  weed, goosegrass, grip grass
Common darter dragonfly (*Sympetrum
  striolatum*)
Common knapweed (*Centaurea nigra*)
Fieldfare (*Turdus pilaris*); a mutation
Goldcrest (*Regulus regulus*)
Redwing (*Turdus iliacus*)

NOVEMBER

Beech (*Fagus*)
Blackthorn (*Prunus spinosa*); fruit: sloes
Field maple (*Acer campestre*)
Hawthorn (*Crataegus* spp.); May, May
  blossom, mother-die, quickthorn
Hazel (*Corylus avellana*)
Sparrowhawk (*Accipiter nisus*)
Spindle (*Euonymus europaeus*)
Wild rose (*Rosa canina*); dog rose

DECEMBER

Lapwing (*Vanellus vanellus*); peewit, teewit,
  teuchitt, green plover
Long-tailed tit (*Aegithalos caudatus*);
  bumbarrel, flying teaspoon, silver-throated
  dasher, long-tailed pie, oven bird, hedge jug;
  zephyr
Roe deer (*Capreolus capreolus*)
Wayfaring tree (*Viburnum lantana*)
Yarrow (*Achillea millefolium*); nosebleed
  plant, sanguinary, old man's pepper, milfoil,
  soldier's woundwort, gordaldo, thousand-
  leaf

JANUARY

Barn owl (*Tyto alba*); golden owl, white owl,
  monkey-faced owl
Hedge-parsley (*Torilis* spp.)
Little egret (*Egretta garzetta*)
Little owl (*Athene noctua*)
Muntjac (*Muntiacus reevesi*)
Seven-spot ladybird (*Coccinella
  septempunctata*); ladybug, red cow, alder
  warbler, lady cow, god's cow, lady's hen
Tawny owl (*Strix aluco*); screech owl, beech
  owl, brown owl; parliament

FEBRUARY

Goat willow (*Salix caprea*); pussy willow
Primrose (*Primula vulgaris*)
Snowdrop (*Galanthus* spp.); candlemas bells,
  fair maids of February, flower of hope
Teasel (*Dipsacus fullonum*)
Wild cherry plum (*Prunus cerasifera*)

MARCH

Common starling (*Sturnus vulgaris*); stuckie,
  starnil, starnie, starn

APRIL

Barn swallow (*Hirundo rustica*)
Blackbird (*Turdus merula*); blackbeep
Dunnock (*Prunella modularis*)
Goldfinch (*Carduelis carduelis*); sheriff, goldie;
  charm
Great tit (*Parus major*)
House sparrow (*Passer domesticus*); spuggy/
  spug, spadger; quarrel, flutter, knot
Jay (*Garrulus glandarius*); scold, party
Oxlip (*Primula elatior*)
Wild garlic (*Allium ursinum*); ramsons
Wood anemone (*Anemone nemorosa*);
  windflower, smellfox

MAY

Bluebell (*Hyacinthoides non-scripta*)
Cow parsley (*Anthriscus sylvestris*); keck, wild-beaked parsley, wild chervil, mother-die
Cowslip (*Primula veris*); cowslop (meaning cowpat)
Hedge bedstraw (*Galium mollugo*)
Lady's bedstraw (*Galium verum*); bedflower
Nightingale (*Luscinia megarhynchos*)
Oxeye daisy (*Leucanthemum vulgare*); dog daisy, moon daisy, moon penny
Pignut (*Conopodium majus*); kippernut, hawknut, earth chestnut, groundnut, earthnut
Tawny mining bee (*Andrena fulva*)
Wild marjoram (*Origanum vulgare*)
Wood avens (*Geum urbanum*)

JUNE

Bee orchid (*Ophrys apifera*)
Borage (*Borago officinalis*)
Breckland thyme (*Thymus serpyllum*)
Common blue butterfly (*Polyommatus icarus*)
Common spotted-orchid (*Dactylorhiza fuchsii*)
Fairy flax (*Linum catharticum*)
Forget-me-nots (*Myosotis* spp.)
Green alkanet (*Pentaglottis sempervirens*)
Hogweed (*Heracleum sphondylium*)
Meadow brown butterfly (*Maniola jurtina*)
Milkwort (*Polygala vulgaris*)
Quaking grass (*Briza* spp.)
Red campion (*Silene dioica*)
Small heath butterfly (*Coenonympha pamphilus*)
Speckled wood butterfly (*Pararge aegeria*)
Small tortoiseshell butterfly (*Aglais urticae*)
Yellow rattle (*Rhinanthus minor*)

JULY

Cinnabar moth (*Tyria jacobaeae*)
Common agrimony (*Agrimonia eupatoria*); church steeples, sticklewort
Common centaury (*Centaurium erythraea*)
Gatekeeper butterfly (*Pyronia tithonus*)

Glow worm (*Lampyris noctiluca*)
Field scabious (*Knautia arvensis*)
Marbled white butterfly (*Melanargia galathea*)
Nightjar (*Caprimulgus europaeus*); moth hawk, night swallow, razor grinder, flying toad
Painted lady butterfly (*Vanessa cardui*)
Ringlet butterfly (*Aphantopus hyperantus*)
Six-spot burnet moth (*Zygaena filipendulae*)
Small skipper butterfly (*Thymelicus sylvestris*)
Southern hawker dragonfly (*Aeshna cyanea*)
White Stork (*Ciconia ciconia*)
Wild carrot (*Daucus carota*); Queen Anne's lace

AUGUST

Acorn barnacle (*Semibalanus balanoides*)
Beadlet anemone (*Actinia equina*)
Chiton (*Lepidochitona cinerea*)
Common blenny (*Lipophrys pholis*); shanny, sea-frog, shan, rocky, bunner
Common periwinkle (*Littorina littorea*)
Common shore crab (*Carcinus maenus*); cast
Common shrimp (*Crangon crangon*)
Plaice (*Pleuronectes platessa*)
Toadflax (*Linaria vulgaris*); butter and eggs, dead men's bones, doggies, false flax, gallwort, impudent lawyer, monkey flower, lion's mouth, snapdragon

SEPTEMBER

Autumn lady's-tresses (*Spiranthes spiralis*)
Bank vole (*Myodes glareolus*)
Blackberry (*Rubus* spp.); bramble
Common toad (*Bufo bufo*); knot, knab, nest
Devil's bit scabious (*Succisa pratensis*)
Eurasian wren (*Troglodytes troglodytes*); chime
Eyebright (*Euphrasia* spp.)
Guelder-rose (*Viburnum opulus*); dogberry, water elder, crampbark, snowball tree
Mason bee (*Osmia* spp.)

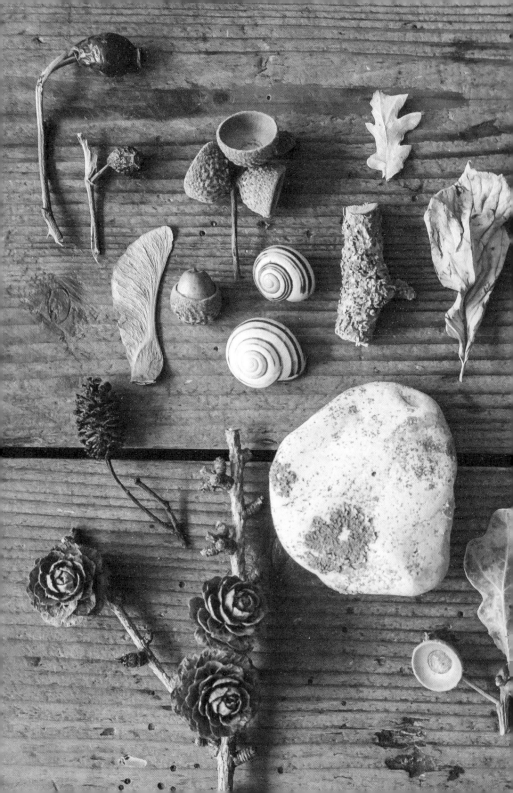

October

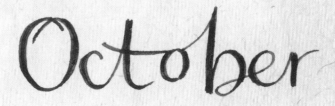

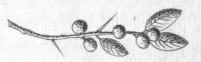

Leaves carpet the ground.
Migrant Thrushes arrive.

I step out of our cottage and the sunlight has that soft, liquid quality that comes as the year turns. The first frost has covered the grass in delicate rime and the early-morning air is sharp and slightly but pleasingly painful in the nose. That redolent, almost mouth-watering smell of leaf mould hangs about the trees and the last of the swallows are leaving. It's autumn.

Annie, our ten-month-old rescue lurcher puppy, is my companion on many of my walks. She is a toffee-coloured, leggy, cheese- and badger-poo-loving, boundless woodland enthusiast, and if I spend too long on my post-breakfast admin she will whimper plaintively, scamper about the living room with her lead in her mouth and poke her snout between my fingers and keyboard to stop my typing, so keen is she for our morning excursions. Once in the wood, I dawdle to watch a ladybird or take a picture of hedge-parsley while she performs her endless busy patrols: checking the tree where the squirrels squabble, sniffing the smeuses (small gaps in the twigs and foliage made by animals) where muntjac deer pass through the hedge. She snaps at leaves as they fall, and she seeks out rotten apples to gnaw on or fox poo with which to anoint herself. She immerses herself in the wood entirely and, I think, regresses to being one of her wolfish ancestors, communing with each smell and merging with it bodily if possible.

This year, October begins with weather that would not be out of place in May or June. It's warm enough for short sleeves and walks in the wood are balmy and sun-drenched. This unseasonal period of sunny weather makes my spirits soar. The sunlight shifts unseen dials of mood-altering neurotransmitters in my brain and I feel cheerful. It is not difficult to rouse myself to my morning walks when the wood is as lovely as this. On the far side of it, the paths between the trees open onto a clearing and here the last of the field scabious are brightening the browning grass with delicate blue-mauve. Knapweed flowers, on which so many butterflies and bees fed and mated earlier in the year, have finished for the season. The knapweed seed heads look like tiny pinecones, with woody scales in a pleasing overlapping pattern. When I am walking I often feel compelled to collect, photograph and record what I find, and sometimes to just take in my environment. Today, I have a strong urge to draw these pinecones, so I gather some to bring home with me.

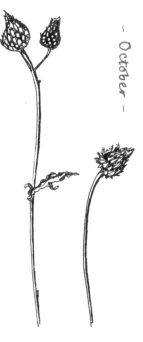

Common
Knapweed

As Annie and I cross the clearing, there are rhythmic glimmers above the mown grass pathways. Dozens of common darter dragonflies have gathered and are seemingly dancing a few inches above the turf. As they dart and wheel, their wings reflect the light and it is an ethereal sight that I wish I could preserve and replay on a winter's day. Their dance is impossible to capture on my phone's camera, so I stop and watch for several minutes, trying to ingrain this encounter in my memory. Later, when I get home, I read about the common darter. This species continues to be active as late as November, favours woodland as a hunting ground for its small insect prey, and can be seen mating in the autumn. I had witnessed an airborne flirtatious quadrille over the seed heads. I wondered where the darters might lay their eggs, then remembered the tiny pond on the edge of the sheep field a few tens of metres from where I saw their display. I file away this dragonfly mating dance as one of the seasonal signposts in the wood: a small October spectacle that I will look out for each year.

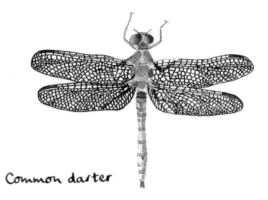

Common darter

It is during October that most trees begin to reabsorb the chlorophyll from their leaves before they fall. As this green pigment, essential for photosynthesis, moves back into the tree it unmasks coloured compounds that have been there all year. Ever-present carotenoids and flavonoids are responsible for the oranges and yellows that appear in woods and parkland at this time of year, and they're joined by the red and occasional pink and purple of anthocyanins whose synthesis begins in autumn. I like the thought that many of the jewel-like colours of spindle, hawthorn, field maple and cherry are there throughout the spring and summer, and that when the weather grows colder and greyer and the fields become drab their colour is revealed.

There is a spot in the wood at the crossroads of two paths where a stand of spindle creates an exquisite but transient patchwork of colour on the woodland floor with their fallen leaves. The colours of spindle leaves hardly seem real during October. Many turn the brightest cerise, some the palest primrose yellow, some a combination of both with a vivid stripe down their centre, and others become almost colourless. As with the sight of the dance of the darters, I want to put this colour into suspended animation so that I might conjure it during the dreary days of January. In a few weeks, colour will be scarce in the countryside. My instinct to gather these bright fallen leaves as I would sea glass or shells on a beach is very strong and I pick some up to take home with me.

When humans explore a new environment and seek out and find resources, the neurotransmitter dopamine is released in the brain, conferring a brief burst of elation: a 'harvest high'. This may be a pathway that was laid down in our hunter-gatherer past. A stand of sea buckthorn covered in berries or a patch of wild strawberries would have boosted the calorific intake of our ancestors, and it would have directly aided their survival to respond positively to the sight of these wild foods, gather the berries and take them back to their shelter. In turn, each incident of foraging that results in edible supplies triggers a reward in the brain and encourages the foraging to become a habit. It is possible that a vestige of this response is what I experience when I gather the spindle leaves. Whatever the evolutionary cause of the positive feelings I gain from gathering them, I know that it is helping to subtly shift the chemical balance in my brain, so I dawdle near the bright carpet and allow the leaves to work their antidepressant spell. The sun is warm. These few minutes in the presence of vivid colours boost my mood in such a tangible way I can almost taste it.

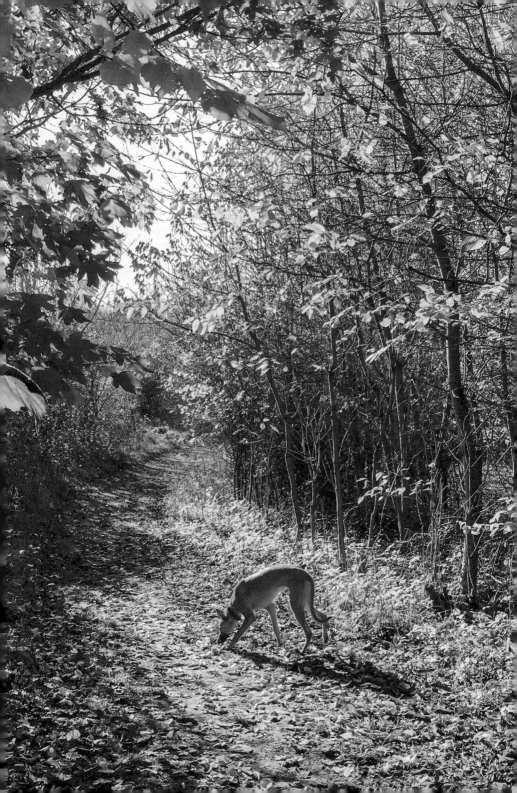

I continue along the woodland paths, ever conscious of Annie's tendency to seek out and roll gleefully in fox and badger poo. On previous occasions when she has finished rolling, she has bounded back to me open-mouthed with dog joy, as though she had doused herself in the rarest, hand-blended Parisian scent and wants me to share in this moment of aromatic luxury. I would prefer to avoid another session scrubbing her down with dog shampoo. Her baths are always followed by several hours when the whiff of wet dog permeates the house and she sulks, cross with my illogical impulse to rid her of the marks and smells of the woods.

She has disappeared for a minute or two, so I stand still, listening for the slight chink of the bone-shaped medallion on her collar. The silence is broken, not by this subtle bell-like sound, but by a series of tiny, high-pitched calls made by something very nearby. I become aware of a small flurry of movement in my peripheral vision and I try to focus on it. A diminutive dark shape is moving among the bare branches of a blackthorn on the edge of the grass path: a bird so tiny that its detail is barely discernible among the tangle of twigs. It is small enough to be obscured in the places where two or three slender branches converge. It flits about, apparently feeding on tiny insects, and does not seem to be aware of me or bothered by my presence. I catch a glimpse of its darkish olive-green plumage. Its head is decorated with a fine yellow stripe, which marks it out as a goldcrest, perhaps one of this year's young.

The goldcrest, along with its cousin the firecrest, is Britain's smallest bird

< Annie in the wood near our cottage

and although common, can be rather tricky to spot as it is well camouflaged among leaves and is usually rather secretive. This individual is so intent on making the most of the prolific insects still present during this warm spell that it doesn't appear to be alarmed by me and continues to dart among the twigs in search of food. The sight of the goldcrest induces a familiar sensation in me. It is the same sudden, giddy, soaring feeling I experienced as a child if I found a minuscule froglet next to my grandad's pond in late summer or a ladybird on a nettle leaf growing near the compost heap. For me, it is better than eating a fine champagne truffle, better even than finding a £10 note down the back of the sofa. It is a new discovery, a small living treasure, something that perhaps only I have seen today.

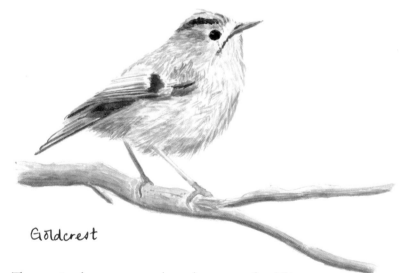

Goldcrest

The turning leaves are not the only source of uplifting colour in the wood in October. The wild roses, hawthorn and sloe bushes are all garlanded with fruit this year. Their branches look like bosky necklaces hung with vegetal beads and it is a beautiful sight. This is a 'berry year' or 'mast year', when the yield of wild fruit is greater than usual and the branches are laden. According to British folklore, woodland trees heavy with berries herald a harsh winter. I like this idea: that the trees can sense the weather to come and provide more food to help the birds to stock up during autumn, increasing their chances of survival. In reality, the large crops of woodland fruit are the result of a warm, dry spring leading to a high rate of pollination, followed by rains in July and August that allowed the resulting substantial embryonic berry crop to swell and develop. But this somewhat less romantic explanation doesn't stop me from being heartened when I think of this prolific natural larder for blackbird, thrush and woodpigeon ready for when the days turn colder.

As the month progresses, I begin to notice flurries of bird activity among the hawthorns on the edge of the village and in the straggly hedge that forms the hem of the wood. Mixed flocks of migrant thrushes, redwings and fieldfares have arrived from Scandinavia, Iceland and Siberia to overwinter in the UK. They touch down just as the woodland fruit crop reaches its peak and they immediately begin to feed on haws, rowan berries and crab apples. Hawthorn bushes full of these charismatic speckle-breasted birds gorging on the berries, or ploughed fields punctuated with them seeking worms in the tilled soil, are a common and to me a precious sight in the Fens during October.

The wood is still rather green, the leaves on many of the trees have yet to turn, and some hedge-parsley and hawkbit

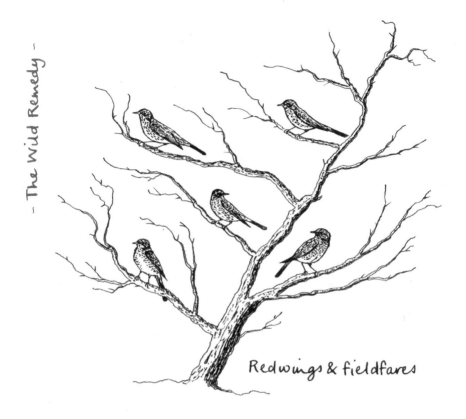

Redwings & fieldfares

plants are still in flower. The markers of late summer are still here, yet along the edge of the mown grass paths I have already begun to notice subtle signs of next spring. Small, delicate fern-like leaves are visible between the grass stems. These are cow parsley seedlings. The seeds of this, my favourite wildflower species, matured during August, fell to the ground and germinated. These tiny new plants will continue to grow until the temperature drops below 4°C; most will survive the winter and flower next May. Alongside the cow parsley seedlings are those of cleavers. This is the plant that children love to pick and stick to their coats (or those of their parents) while out on walks. Its colloquial names include sticky bobs, goosegrass and sticky weed, and the slender stalks of these new seedlings are punctuated with tiny rosettes of delicate leaves along their length. These new plants will be present throughout the winter, growing slowly provided the temperature stays several degrees above freezing. They are the tangible beginnings of next spring, already here in the wood. I find this thought very cheering and I vow to come and peep at them on days when I succumb to winter gloom.

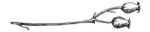

As each year passes here in the Fens, I learn more about the wildlife and particularly the botany that lives near our cottage. If I find a plant I am unfamiliar with, I try to learn its name, find out where it fits among the families of plant life I already know, and in this way I grow more familiar with this place and feel I know and understand it a little more. Today, I find a small, delicate flower in the wood that I don't recognize. It grows on the edge of the clearing, its roots in chalky soil and its leaves in patches of dappled shade. It is delicately beautiful: a slender stem around 15 cm tall topped with small, chalice-shaped, pinkish-mauve flowers. Its petals are fine and narrow, and when the flowers have finished they are replaced by tiny powder puffs of soft seeds, like those of members of the dandelion family. I assume that it's a variety of hawkbit and I come home to pore over my reference books and search the internet. I cannot see any plants that match it among my books: their flowers are all yellow and most are showier than those of this species. I google British hawkbits and still no luck.

Then, while flicking through Keble Martin, a smallish pink-mauve flower catches my eye on Plate 44: the same page and family as the common daisy and wild asters. I have found it: blue fleabane or *Erigeron acer*. Keble Martin's painting captures the simple beauty of this plant perfectly. It's new to me and now I'm keen to see more specimens so I return to the wood to draw and paint it. The soothing process of taking up my pencil and paintbrush and making simple marks on paper that mimic the shape of this rather humble flower distracts me from nagging, rumbling thoughts.

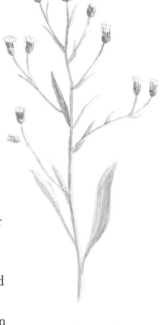

Blue fleabane

Later in the month I am feeling tired and rather low. In winter a transient depression called Seasonal Affective Disorder (SAD) can descend due to the lack of sunlight, which, in turn, can affect levels of serotonin in the brain. It is thought that some people are more sensitive to the effects of less bright sunlight in winter and that in these individuals neurotransmitter levels shift more markedly, resulting in lethargy and low mood between November and March. Between 20 and 30 per cent of the UK population suffers from SAD in some form. I experience this seasonal sadness each year and I fear it may be beginning to brew in my neurons, like dismal tea. For me, spending time near the sea is particularly effective at fending off mental darkness so I travel to Kent, meet up with my friend Helen and we drive to the pebble-covered promontory of Dungeness.

On difficult days I often reach for *Derek Jarman's Garden*. I find Howard Sooley's superb photographs visually soothing and I'm enchanted by the way Jarman describes taming the shingle that grew around his Dungeness home of Prospect Cottage. The result was a parched but exquisite patch of maritime plants, flint pebbles, metal and driftwood that he found on the strandline and added to the garden. Jarman corralled the local wild botany, added rusted and rounded artefacts thrown up by the sea, and made a few square metres of rugged yet sublime planting: a place that is arid yet green. I long to visit Prospect Cottage but am also on a mission to see the lichen heath that grows on the shingle: a complex microworld of lichens and hardy pioneer plant species no more than 4 cm high.

Lichens are one of the only groups of organisms that can tolerate the lack of moisture on the Dungeness pebble dunes. Each is a symbiotic colony of microorganisms containing both a fungus and an alga, sometimes joined by a bacterium, and they form delicate tapestries in the hollows of the shingle. The aqua greys of *Cladonia mitis* and *Hypogymnia physodes*, the mustard yellow of *Xanthoria parietina*, and the pale chartreuse of *Flavoparmelia caperata* are muted and beautiful.

Helen and I wonder at these tiny, hardy forests, take pictures of the bleached wooden fishing boats sitting on the shingle and linger in the Prospect Cottage garden looking at rosehips, horned poppy seed heads and little pebble henges. We eat fish and chips outside a pub looking at the sea and talk for several hours. I'm fortified by what I see on this gargantuan, ancient pile of pebbles and by Helen's company. This brief trip has allayed my lurking low mood. The SAD is at bay for now, but

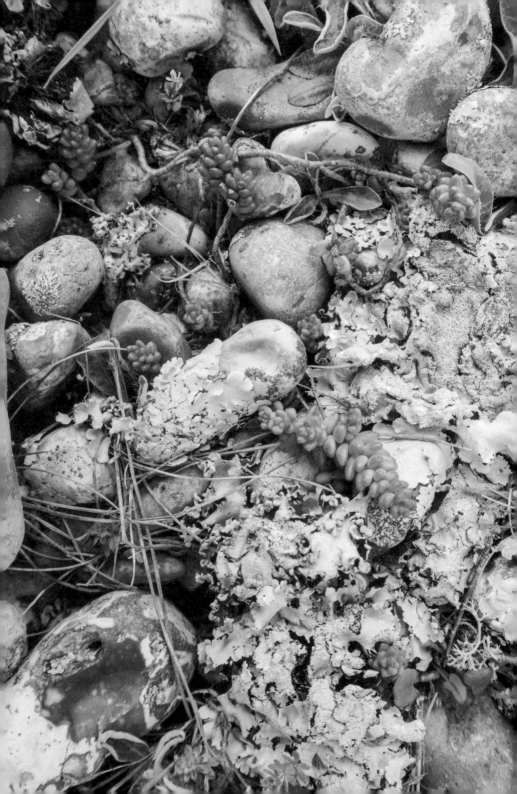

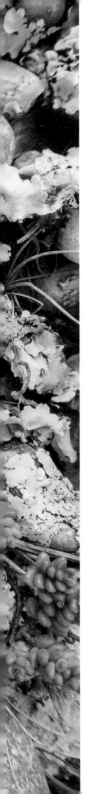

with two more months until midwinter, the sun will continue to shift away from the northern hemisphere, taking my motivation and energy with it. I long for a more prolonged dose of Dungeness but must return home.

‹ Lichen heath at Dungeness

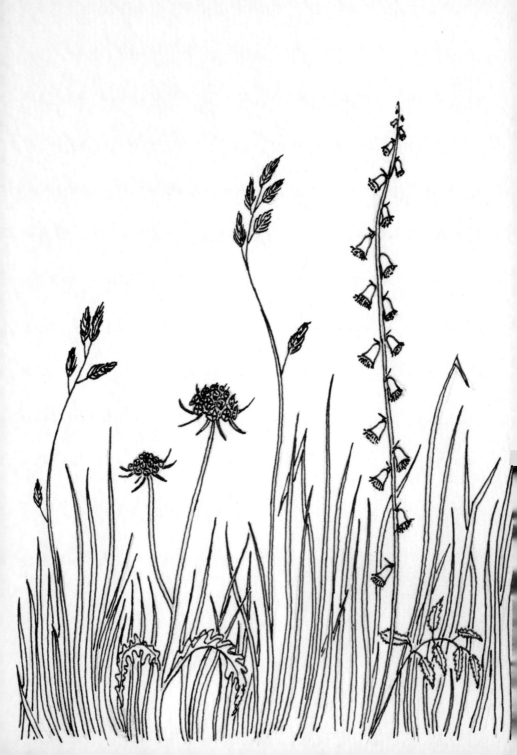

November

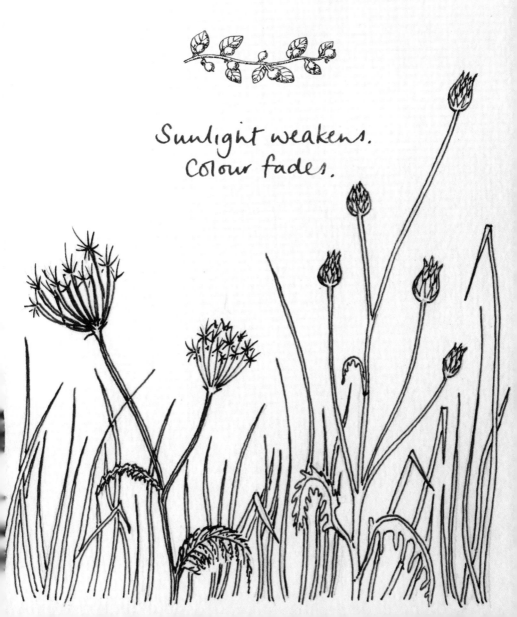

Sunlight weakens.
Colour fades.

I confess I can harbour resentment towards autumn for its chicanery. It often begins with a hint that, this year, winter will not arrive. 'Look,' it seems to say, 'hedge-parsley is still in flower, it's as warm as June.' I know its tricks. A slight atmospheric shift and Indian summer gives way to thickly clouded skies and penetrating, joy-stealing cold. It is these first hints of the sunless, colourless weeks to come when I can lose heart.

Each year I approach late autumn and winter as though I'm scaling a mountain: a seemingly insurmountable peak that looms and can drain my entire body of vitality. The foothills can be daunting and I wish I could tunnel through the bloody thing with the giant rock-gnawing drill that carved out the Channel tunnel. I long to circumvent the months to come and pop up in late February like a five-foot ten-inch mole, just in time to see blackthorn buds swelling. The northern hemisphere has shifted away from the sun and it takes my verve with it. If I succumb to the inexorable downward pull of SAD, it will be almost impossible to free myself from the sofa.

It's in November that each walk I take becomes crucial. Whatever the sky might be doing, ten minutes spent in the wood can alter the balance of the neurotransmitters in my brain that will help shift the tone of my thoughts and work to keep me going. If the sun does emerge, then that dose of mood-shifting brain chemicals is even stronger, and if I spot a jay, some hedge-parsley or a speckled wood butterfly basking on a leaf, then the gentle nature-spotters' high I experience means that the walk is even more medicinal and I can return home feeling almost ebullient, in defiance of the approaching winter.

I am a colour-seeker. As winter nears, my urge to

encounter as many brights as possible in the wood and hedgerows becomes almost feverish. Despite the sky being suffused with grey, I know that there is still colour in the wood, so I set out to find some. Last month, the spindle leaves lifted my spirits.

Beech

This month their berries ripen and the emergent pinks and oranges are almost psychedelic in their vividness. Meanwhile, the field maple leaves, miniature versions of their sycamore cousins, have turned gold, beech has become a glowing copper, and sloes are indigo with a delicate covering of frosty bloom. I covet all of it, as I did last month, but now these sights are increasingly scarce and my desire to hold on to them, to *own* a little of them,

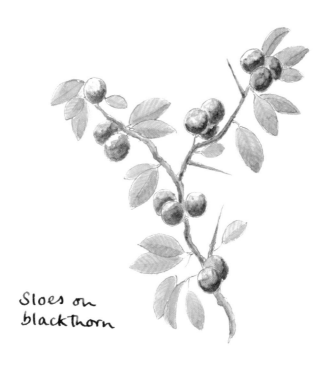

Sloes on
blackthorn

becomes more acute; I want to stuff all this colour hungrily into my eyes and pockets while it lasts. I gather a little of everything, as though it's a botanical pick-and-mix, and bring it home to photograph.

Liquid blue skies follow a cold clear night. The ground has hardened and patches of frost lie in the shadows. It's easier to walk on days like this: the sun lures me outdoors. In the wood many of the leaves that fell last month have been browned and softened by ice, mud and several kinds of trampling feet. Several nights of frost have burgled the wood of much of its vibrancy. I mourn for the lost colour but there are still a few brights to be found. I walk the path that skirts the clearing in the wood. Most of the cherry leaves that were so vivid last month are on the ground, their colour fading, but through the branches I spot a patch of brilliant yellow and push through the trees to reach it. There, in a place where bee and heath orchids flower in June, is a field maple in its November outfit. This tree is a cousin of Japanese acers and a diminutive relative of the maples that are feted for their autumn colour in New England at this time of year. Its leaves are a truly stunning hue: brighter than primroses, as vivid as lemons. As I stand and gaze, the low November sun illuminates each leaf from behind and this natural spectacle is as beautiful as any stained-glass window. The sunlight is itself rather golden at this time of year due to the relative angle of the sun and northern hemisphere, and to the light travelling through more atmosphere before it reaches the tree, so these little maple leaves seem to blaze. I let my eyes soak up the light and colour for some time and I'm left feeling almost rapturous. As I return to the clearing I search for the little glossy rosettes of bee orchid leaves, but I fail to spot them.

Nature finds from the wood near our cottage ›
and corresponding drawings

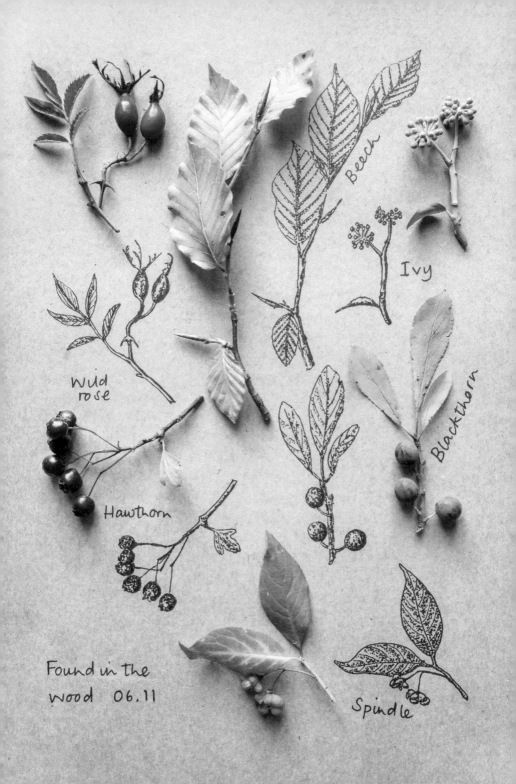

Beech

Ivy

Wild
rose

Blackthorn

Hawthorn

Found in the
wood 06.11

Spindle

I know they are there, yet they seem adept at hiding among the grass and fronds of yarrow and wild carrot.

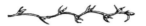

For observers of nature there can sometimes seem to be a sort of bus-like phenomenon with wildlife encounters and I experience this midway through November. I haven't seen any sparrowhawks for many months, then I see two in a week. Annie and I are deep in the wood one morning when a sparrowhawk manifests itself at the edge of my vision. The sighting is fleeting, two seconds at most and little more than a darkish retinal blur, leaving me questioning whether I saw the hawk at all. It is a feathered wraith, flying at speed through the trees just a few metres from me, and I catch a glimpse of its horizontally barred grey-and-cream breast feathers. As it travels it flexes its wings and effortlessly shifts the angle of its trajectory to avoid collisions with trunks and branches. The alacrity of these aerial manoeuvres speaks of a humblingly accurate gyroscope and navigation system. The sparrowhawk harbours a small but very powerful prey-seeking computer in its head.

The second sparrowhawk appears while I sit in a queue of traffic in Suffolk. There are stubble fields and hedgerows to either side of the road and a flurry of distant movement catches my attention. The hawk appears over a hedge with just centimetres between the tip of its wings and the twigs below, and soars down into the field to skim over the stumps of barley stalks with rapid and regular wing-beats. It flies over the cars, continues its path across the field on the other side of the road, makes an aerial leap over the hedge beyond and flits out of sight. It is like a little death jet with murderous intent upon finches, pigeons and starlings. This sighting is a giddy highlight in an otherwise grey, mundane day. The stealth of sparrowhawks, their steely purposefulness, elusiveness and tendency to rise up behind hedges, walls and between trees, mean that when I see one I experience a more intense thrill than if I see a kestrel hovering above a verge. In the unspoken raptor-spotting Top Trumps, sparrowhawk trounces kestrel.

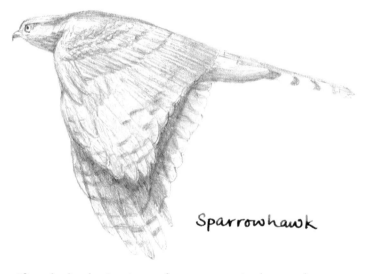

Sparrowhawk

If we don't take Annie out for a scamper in the woods at least once a day, her excess energy leaks out as bouts of curve-tailed frenzied dashing up and down the stairs or plaintive songs in a comical canine soprano, sung to the crow she sees through the living room window, which often struts about on the village green. Annie is the orange dog who draws me out on days when the black dog sinks its teeth into my neurons and bites down hard. If she becomes frustrated at the lateness of her walk she will vent her ire on certain inanimate objects that take on the role of nemesis at such moments. She becomes particularly vexed with the wooden hearth brush, which over time has lost its bristles and then its handle, leaving a gnawed stump. Pencils are also her arch-enemies when she is keen to get to the wood. On a day when a phone call kept me from taking her out at the usual time I found the splintered remains of my favourite Derwent HB in the corner.

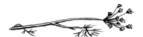

It's the third week of November and the weather is dank. For me, there's a constant mental battle between what my depression would like me to do on days like this and the activities I know will lift it. My overwhelming urge to stay in the house and barely move comes from my susceptibility to the lower levels of bright sunlight in late autumn and winter, causing my energy levels to falter. This is combined with the long-term effects of family anxieties and pressures, leading to raised stress levels, but I know the balance of both can be shifted if I prise myself away from my cosy nest and venture among trees and plants.

I manage to get out, despite the lowering skies. Annie is gleeful and we take our usual route through the wood. There are several crossways among the paths as we walk and one of my favourite spots is the place where the path onto the clearing intersects with a route that skirts the wood. In spring and summer the clearing is a riot of wildflowers: knapweed, hawkbits, scabious, wild carrot, grasses, goat's-beard, blue fleabane and, in a very few spots, bee and common spotted-orchids. The path that runs along the edge of the wood is the place where I sometimes find ladybirds hibernating in winter among the seed heads. On one side of the path there is a tall rough hedge of blackthorn that is a popular spot for winter thrushes and bullfinches, and on the other side is a stand of young beech trees.

At the place where this path crosses our main route through the wood there is a log bench surrounded by hawthorn and wild roses, and a young walnut tree stands on the corner. This is one of my favourite places to sit, especially when the sun is strong enough to warm my face. Opposite is a mature hazel, the third corner is a tangle of roses beneath cherry trees, and on the fourth are the spindle bushes, whose leaves I collected last month.

As we reach the intersection of paths, something catches my eye: small points of pale grey-green on the hazel tree. I move my head to look more closely, and see that they are bright against the background of grey skies and skeletal trees. Paperclip-sized embryonic catkins have emerged. They are the hazel tree's male flowers and will continue to elongate slowly between now and February, when they will open to release pollen, to be caught by the tiny cerise star-shaped female flowers.

There are several small sights that I seek out during the darker months. They're subtle botanical beacons: heartening signs that reassure me of spring's eventual arrival. These immature catkins are just such a sign, as are the delicate

Hawthorn

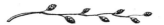

cow parsley and cleavers seedlings that began to emerge last month. Spring *will* come; nights *will* shorten, my thoughts *will* feel lighter again. I dawdle near the hazel for a while. I notice Annie sniffing with great interest at a dropping of some kind nearby and whisk her away before she has time to smear herself with a terrible stench.

Hazel catkins

In the last week of November I can feel hints of the dragging greyness that can dominate my thoughts and entire outlook. When I dip this low, prolonged walks are necessary, or failing that, time spent by the sea, and my mind returns to last month's trip to Dungeness. Once again, I'm drawn to the coast and, despite the penetrating cold and threat of rain, I drive to Essex on a repeated pilgrimage. Walton-on-the-Naze is a seaside town that appears to be stuck in a previous decade, its streets lined with chintzy cafes and old-fashioned hardware stores. Much as I love a day of ice creams, sandcastles and penny falls, today I'm aiming for the Naze tower and the shore to the north of the main beach.

I descend the steps from the Naze visitor car park, start northwards along the concrete walkway towards the beach, climb down onto the sands and make my way towards the cliff. Just here it is a well-defined layer cake of geological eras. Standing in front of this vertical timeline, I can see a thin strip of stones just beneath the grasses at the top of the cliff. These are gravels deposited by the Thames around 600,000 years ago. This idea is captivating: the ancestral

Thames, pre-dating even the very earliest settlement that
eventually gave rise to London's vast sprawl, meandered
across Essex and deposited these pebbles. My mind capsizes
slightly. The Thames has been flowing for more than half a
million years and when this layer was set down hominids
were just beginning to evolve into Neanderthals. There is
archaeological evidence for the earliest signs of cooking that
is contemporary with these Thames gravels. I could easily
lose hours standing and thinking about this, but I'm in
search of fossils in the lower layers of the cliff.

Beneath the Thames gravels is an amber-coloured sandy
formation called the Red Crag. Two million years ago,
Essex was covered by a cool sea, teeming with marine life
that accumulated on the seabed and built up shell-rich
dunes along the shore. These sands became the Red Crag.
It is reddish orange due to iron pyrite washing into it from
the basal layer of the cliff and oxidizing once there.

A little lower is an area of Red Crag that has fallen away
and, even before I have drawn near, I can see more exposed
shells. Here and there are fossilized whelks among the sand
grains, and I fall on them gleefully. These are specimens of
Neptunea contraria, an extinct species whose shells spiral in
the opposite direction to modern whelks, and almost every
other species of gastropod. They are easy to find and apart
from a slightly rusty appearance from being in the Red Crag
sands they look as though they were washed up not long ago,
yet they are several million years old. For the second time
today I feel awestruck by these glimpses into a previous era.

I clamber back down onto the beach. Here the lowest
layer of the cliff merges with the sand. This is the 54-million-
year-old London Clay formation, a soft bluish deposit that
represents a period of Britain's history when the climate

was subtropical and sharks and turtles swam in warm seas. Fossils of birds, crustaceans, mammals such as horses and whales, and the fruit and seeds of trees can also be found in the London Clay, and all may be found on the beach. I regard these sands as a vast cabinet of curiosities or *wunderkammer*.

As I begin my search, rain starts to fall, a persistent wind whips up the beach from the sea and it is horribly cold. This sort of weather would normally force me back to my car, but I'm determined to continue my search and my eyes scan the sand as I walk. Within minutes I find the tooth of a *Striatolamia* shark. Elongated, wickedly sharp and with a dark sheen, it came from the mouth of a huge cartilaginous fish that lived around 54 million years ago.

When I return home, I lay out my discoveries from Walton-on-the-Naze alongside my collection of modern and fossilized mollusc shells. As I display and examine shells, botanical finds or fossils, my mind enters a state similar to that triggered by painting or kneading bread dough: my mental clamour is quietened and a calm descends. I am generating smallish temporary displays, short-lived museums curated by and for me, and the making of them soothes, lifts gloom and adds to the satisfaction I felt on finding these small items. I'm curious about the mental pathways linked to sorting and arranging, and wonder whether they hark back to the processing of leaves, berries, seeds, nuts and shellfish that our ancestors may have undertaken after foraging trips. Investigating this link would require a sizeable research budget and a small team of archaeologists and neuroscientists. All I know is that neatly laying out the things I find, or 'knolling' as it is known on social media, mitigates stress and leaves me gently uplifted.

Fossils found at Walton-on-the-Naze

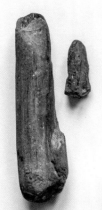

Pyritised twigs from the 56-49m. year old London Clay layer. During this era Britain's climate was subtropical.

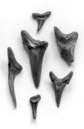

Striatolamia sharks' teeth from the London Clay. 50 million years ago sharks & turtles swam off the Essex coast.

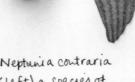

Aequipecten opercularis or queen scallop, found in the Red Crag. 1.8-3m years old.

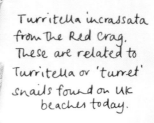

Turritella incrassata from the Red Crag. These are related to Turritella or 'turret' snails found on UK beaches today.

Neptunia contraria (left) a species of whelk that lived around 2m. years ago. Its spiral twists the opposite way to that of modern whelks (right)

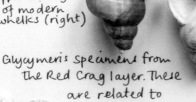

Glycymeris specimens from the Red Crag layer. These are related to modern dog cockles.

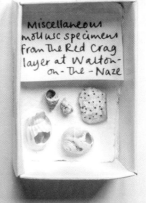

Miscellaneous mollusc specimens from the Red Crag layer at Walton-on-the-Naze

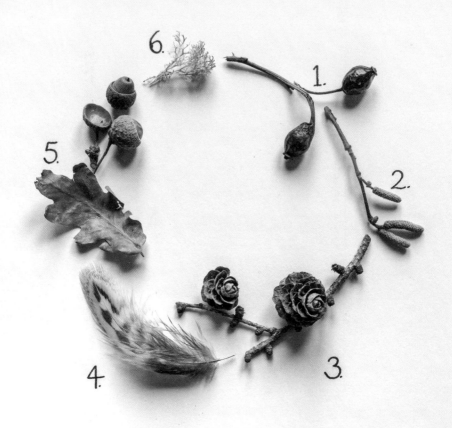

1. Wild rosehips from
   the village wood.
2. Catkins from the
   village wood.
3. Larch cones from a
   wood near Wareham.
4. Tawny owl feather
   from Bradfield woods.
5. Oak leaf and acorns
   from near Upware.
6. Cladonia mitis from
   Dungeness.

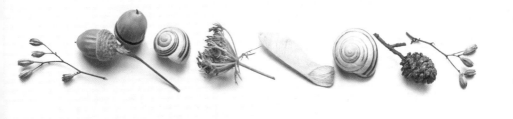

December

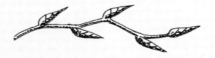

The shortest days.
Starlings gather.

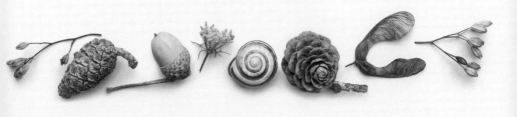

We have left the last of the balmy days behind and ahead lies cold and Christmas. The pleasant twinkliness and food-based indulgence of the festive season does little to assuage the bleakness that can descend upon my mind in December. I know that the next few months will be the toughest to surmount. My levels of serotonin and dopamine have never been tested, but my entire outlook shifts, my verve scarpers and I feel certain that these changes are caused by shifts in neuronal chemistry between December and February.

When my mind enters this state its very ability to respond to beautiful sights seems to diminish. The decreased intensity of sunlight in the northern hemisphere is not only the trigger for this neuronal change, but also leads to changes in the local botany. It is the *combination* of the stronger sunlight entering my eye and the colourful sights of primrose, scabious, hawkbit, cherry blossom, poppy and the intense greens of foliage that serve to make my mood significantly more ebullient in spring and summer. As the sunlight weakens, so the flowers fade and colour drains from the landscape. My synapses are dealt a doubly stultifying blow.

It is during these weeks that it can become difficult to move. The depression feeds on itself and grows stronger through stillness; as a result the effort needed to leave the house can become Herculean. The cycle of feeling low, remaining stationary, the resulting droop in mood, staying even more still and the inexorable downward spiral, can feel as impossible to halt as the shift in season that triggers it. I can feel myself becoming more sessile, like a morose limpet, and I know I must find a foothold to prevent me from succumbing to this dark, vertiginous, slippery-walled hole.

I have to force myself to continue to take Annie for walks. The grasses have faded and recent rainfall has left them lying in collapsed, frost-browned clumps in the clearing. They remind me of so many discarded soggy wigs and have a hint about them of a certain American president's baffling coiff. Wild carrot and yarrow seed heads have faded to dun, the last of the hawkbits have ceased to flower and the path around this meadow-ish patch of land presents a muddy, drab prospect. I am beginning to long for vivid chlorophyll greens, but fortunately rosehips have not yet succumbed to ice crystals, so here and there are pinpricks of vermillion. The path loops around the clearing and on the other side is a dense patch of hawthorn and wayfaring tree. This low scrubby patch of wood is a favourite place for birdlife and I have heard the calls of green woodpecker, blackcap, wren, chiffchaff, blackbird, chaffinch and robin here during the warmer months. There are still a very few hawthorn berries or haws on the lichen-encrusted branches and I stop to examine them. They're the colour of claret, each with a star-shaped scar, marking the last vestige of the flower that opened in May, was pollinated and gave rise to this small fruit. They are a cheering sight and I picked hundreds of haws here in August to infuse in gin. Hawthorn is related to the rose family and the resulting liqueur tastes of Turkish delight and of heady, scented summer. The contrast

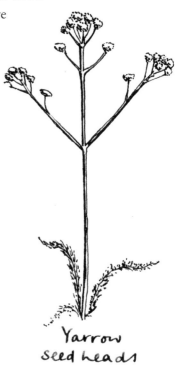

Yarrow
Seed heads

between the deep wine-coloured berries and the subtle blue-grey and yellow-green filigrees of the lichens is beautiful and I'm grateful for these colours today.

We make our way towards home and as we pass through the blackthorn-dense centre of the wood, near the spot where I saw the goldcrest in October, a pattern of tiny birdcalls seems to emanate from more than one spot among the upper branches. The sounds are moving and I try to pinpoint their source. A flock of long-tailed tits is travelling along the tops of the blackthorns, but they are not flying together in a group as starlings or finches might; instead they're performing an ornithological relay, spread in a line several metres long. The leading bird makes a quick swooping flight of half a metre or so and the one behind it does the same, followed by the next. They take turns in their flight and as the bird behind catches up, so the one in front moves again. They call as they go: sharp, high-pitched, breathy whistles that are emitted in time with the movement. I marvel at this coordinated method of journeying, like a mobile cat's cradle. I have witnessed it before along the Devil's Dyke in Cambridgeshire, an ancient Anglo-Saxon earthwork near our cottage, and in Bradfield Woods near Bury St Edmunds, and perhaps its purpose is to evade or confuse sparrowhawks as the long-tailed tits move between trees where they roost and feed.

The long-tailed tits' swagged flight lines lend them an air of jauntiness. I'm anthropomorphizing, but they look as though they're enjoying their looping, flitting route through the wood and, despite the nagging bleakness in my mind, I, too, enjoy this small wild sight and the welcome distraction it offers. Annie doesn't notice them. I realize that while I was gazing at the birds she had discovered a

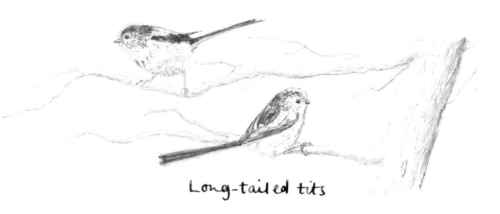

Long-tailed tits

malodorous, feathered dead something on the edge of the path and wolfed it down before I could discourage her. I worry about its possible effects on her innards as we return to the cottage.

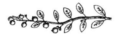

One afternoon I drive out of our village and head across the Fenland countryside towards the villages of Upware and Wicken. This road has so much subsidence that in places driving along it feels like being in the carriage of a rollercoaster. The ricketiness of the road adds to the feeling of otherworldliness that descends on me when I spend time in the Fens. This is a 400-year-old landscape, formed when this part of East Anglia was drained in the seventeenth century by harnessing a combination of English and Dutch knowledge. Prior to the drainage, these fields were submerged and livings were made from cutting reed, hunting waterfowl, fishing and barge-bound transport. We live not far from the sandy-soiled area of East Anglia called the Brecklands, meaning 'broken lands'. The horizon is dotted with the characteristic maritime pines of the Brecks, along with alders, willows and stands of reeds. This is agricultural land, which means that in places there is a green sterility where biodiversity is quashed by fertilizers and pesticides, but the arable fields are interspersed with islands of fen that have been reclaimed by the National Trust. The Fen Vision project plans to acquire a continuous thread of countryside between Wicken and the edge of Cambridge and to allow it to revert to the waterland of five centuries ago. On the outskirts of our village is a parcel of land that is part of this scheme: a stretch of wild grassland with a small reservoir, where large flocks of starlings sometimes roost, where hobbies snatch dragonflies from the air in summer and where ghostly short-eared owls drift in from Scandinavia and spend the winter hunting among the frosted grasses.

As I traverse the Fen I spot a flock of birds in the distance and drive closer. At this time of day it is common to see smallish flocks of starlings wheeling over the Fen before they roost, but these birds are larger and they make extravagant swerving lines in the air. I pull the car over and rummage for binoculars. The blunt shapes of their wings and their pale undersides mark them out as lapwings, also known as peewits. I have been enthralled by this species of bird since I first saw them as a child through a car window as several stood in a ploughed field by the side of the M6 in Cheshire. It was their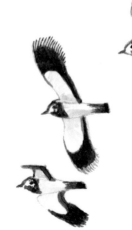

iridescent teal and black wings and flamboyant feathered fascinator that made me incredulous when I first saw them by the motorway. I thought they looked exotic, as though they belonged in a far-off land; they were birds-of-paradise in a conurbation. Their wheeling flight patterns and plangent, almost metallic-sounding call with hints of ventriloquy make the lapwing even more beguiling. It is on the UK's red list of birds of conservation concern, because the numbers of breeding pairs have declined drastically in the last quarter-century, so to see a flock of a hundred or more individuals

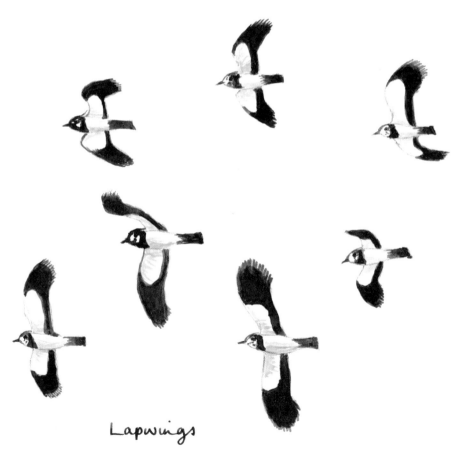

Lapwings

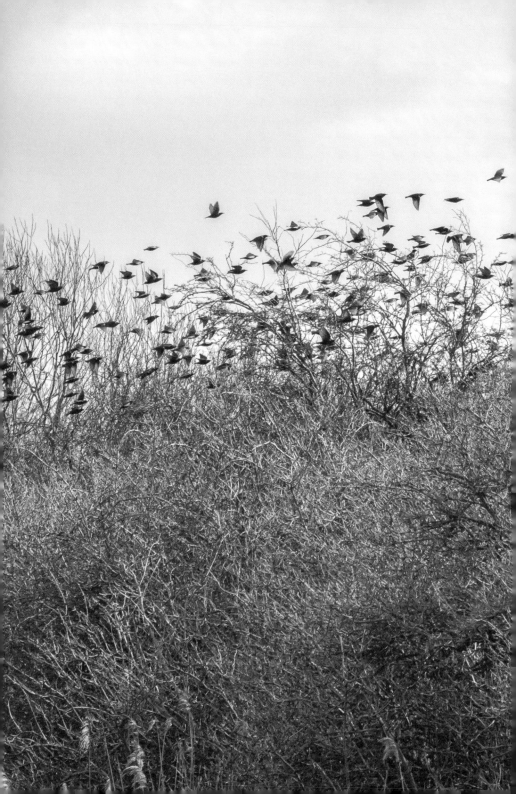

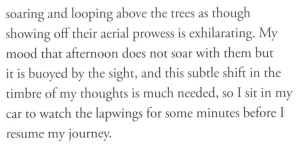

soaring and looping above the trees as though showing off their aerial prowess is exhilarating. My mood that afternoon does not soar with them but it is buoyed by the sight, and this subtle shift in the timbre of my thoughts is much needed, so I sit in my car to watch the lapwings for some minutes before I resume my journey.

This species has declined in number since the beginning of the twentieth century, but here in the Fens, rough grazing, spring-sown crops and unimproved grassland form a mosaic of habitats that encourage successful lapwing broods.

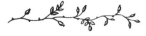

It is the 21st of December, the winter solstice, and the hours of sunlight have reached their annual minimum. The darkness of the days has pinned me down and the impervious granite mountain of winter is sitting on my mind. Life begins to feel like wading through viscous mud and each day is utterly exhausting. These are some of the hardest weeks of the year. My cocktail of neurotransmitters seems to be missing crucial ingredients that confer mental energy and an ability to experience pleasure, and this has been exacerbated by the shortening days. I know that it's likely that the levels of dopamine and perhaps serotonin are low in my brain just now, and I wonder if there are other neuronal messengers or components that we have not yet discovered, which also fall away as SAD tightens its grip.

Making myself move and, if I am truthful, live,

‹ A small fenland murmuration of starlings

takes all the effort I can muster, so it is during midwinter that I let myself off the walking hook, and I have found that driving about the Fenland countryside in the car can benefit my mind almost as much as setting foot in the wood. I know it is not ecologically sound to take a drive with no real destination in mind, and guilt gnaws at me, but I also know that if I see some skeletal winter trees against an ashen sky, catch a glimpse of a kestrel hovering above a verge or spot a small gaggle of bustly partridges in a field, there will be a subtle yet immensely welcome shift in my mind and it will feel like a few starlings lifting from their roost.

I drive towards Dullingham, a small village between our house and Haverhill. It's a road lined with fallow and cropped fields, pockets of woodland and unkempt hedgerows. I have steered this route hundreds of times at night, when my mind has been wracked with the aftermath of illnesses or the incessant onslaught of difficult days. I have seen owls as I've driven: tawny, little and barn. I've seen hares, crouching in a scrape or running at full speed parallel to the road, appearing to race the car. Sometimes mice or voles dart across the carriageway in what seems like a terrible panic. A stoat or weasel are rarer sights, zooming across the tarmac like murderous hairy cigars.

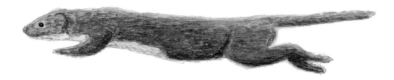

Weasel

There is a patch of higher ground between our village and
Dullingham: a low plateau covered in ploughed fields. Here
the road is lined with young ash trees and sometimes a barn
owl sits in one of them at dusk. As I drive I become aware
of a collection of dark shapes against the winter wheat and
glance over to see deer moving in the opposite direction to
my journey. I pull the car over and can see that one is a buck
and has short but striking antlers, and that they have quite
large oval patches of white fur on their rumps. They are roe
deer and the sight of them striding across the field is joyous.
This is an ancient scene, something that will have been
witnessed for centuries. Although small for a deer, the roe is
one of the largest mammals in Britain and there is a group of
wild individuals quite near to where I live. Something about
the regal deportment of the buck, and the way the three
individuals are walking in a line like woodland hieroglyphics,
makes this a special sighting. The deer make me think of
this land of ours, how we have ravaged it with modern
farming methods, with fertilizers and with insecticides, how
we have grubbed up woods and water meadows in order to
grow more food and maximize profit. I think of the plight
of the bees, the decimation of pollinator populations, and
how that has threatened the survival of so many of our
bird species, yet here are these roe deer walking across this
field of winter wheat shoots. It's a privilege to see them,
yet I feel ambivalent. I yearn for a glimpse of sixteenth-
century England where their ancestors lived. I long to be in
countryside where the numbers of returning nightingales and
cuckoos do not diminish each year and where flocks of corn
buntings still make rich livings on farmland. I am glad I saw
the deer and of course this sighting helped my mind, as each
one does, but as I drive away I feel troubled.

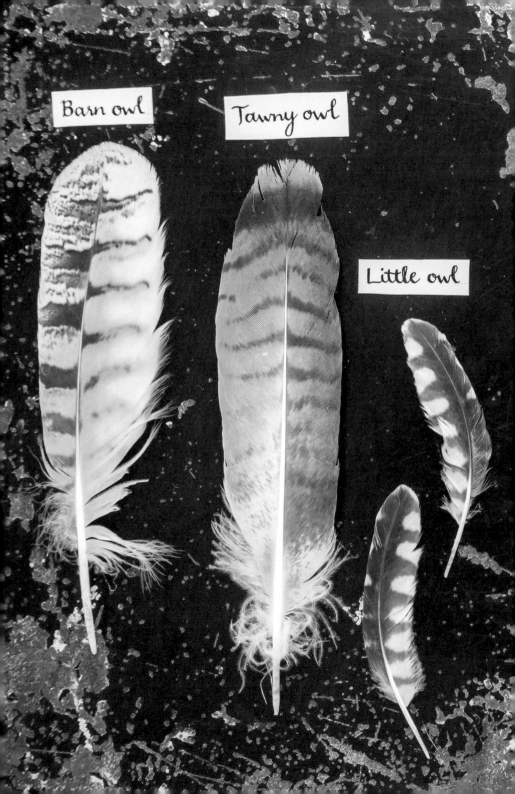

Barn owl

Tawny owl

Little owl

January

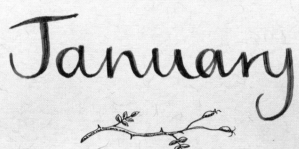

Ladybirds sleep.
Snowdrop shoots emerge.

Kestrel

Great spotted
woodpecker

Pheasant

I always feel some relief at the arrival of the New Year. The weeks that stretch out between Christmas and the beginning of spring can be the darkest, both meteorologically and neurologically, yet the 1st of January is a mental milestone of sorts. Around half of winter has passed, I've got through it without succumbing to depression's darkest pit, and with that heartening thought comes a few days of a fresher feeling, a lighter mood.

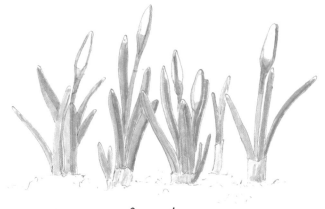

Snowdrops

As Annie and I walk up to the wood on one of the first days of the year, I know that snowdrops are emerging in the patch of land owned by a neighbour to the left of the path. I peer through the fence but the place where the snowdrops usually appear is too far from where I am standing to be able to see whether I'm looking at blades of grass or the new shoots. There's a small gate through the hedge leading to this fenced-off area, and I steal through. There they are, just a few centimetres tall, unfeasibly verdant and juicy-looking. This is a watershed find in my year: the shoots of the earliest flowers. It is like the first curry after weeks without that spicy warmth, the first cup of tea drunk outside in the tentative March sun. These snowdrops are the botanical equivalent of *Star Wars Episode IV: A New Hope*.

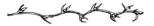

I drive home from Cambridge fairly early one evening. My eldest daughter is with me and we are feeling content after a shopping trip followed by a delicious burger. As I slow down at the threshold of the village we notice a slight movement near the hedge. 'What's a child doing waiting for a bus in the dark?' I think, but it isn't a child. It is a muntjac deer standing next to the bus stop signpost as though it is waiting for the number ten to Newmarket. My headlights startle the deer only slightly, so that it pushes its way into the hedge behind the bus stop, enough to hide its head and front quarters but leaving its tan rump sticking out. There it stands surrounded by twigs, bum protruding but fancying itself out of sight. It reminds me of my youngest daughter covering her eyes when she was very small and thinking this made her invisible when we played hide-and-seek.

I wonder if this might be the same muntjac that had woken both daughters up each night for several weeks back in the autumn, by trotting onto the village green in front of our cottage and barking loudly and raspily to potential mates in the early hours. Or it could be the father of the baby muntjac I saw with its mother in the spring of last year, in the same patch of fenced-off woodland where I saw the snowdrops emerging. I had been walking up to the wood with our first dog, Minnie, who by then was

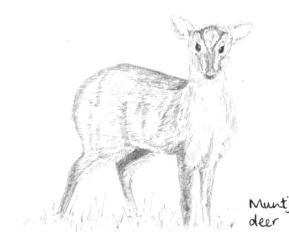

Muntjac
deer

very elderly, and I heard a sort of high-pitched peeping
sound just beyond the fence and among the trees to my
left. There was a loud rustling and an adult muntjac leaped
away from the fence with a movement like a slightly stout
antelope. She turned and with her eyes on me she called
gruffly. Something scurried towards her from beneath some
brambles: her conker-coloured miniature, the size of a small
cat. The baby muntjac joined its mother and they scarpered
through a straggly hedge of hawthorn and out of sight.

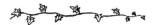

Soon after my snowdrop sighting, the weather and the
landscape become resolutely wet, cold and colourless.
Daylight hours are still short, light levels are low, mood-
buoying neurotransmitters ebb away, energy levels slump.
After several days of this weather it becomes difficult to
move. I cower in the cottage, my mind weighed down by
a blanket of malaise and immobility. I long for the sun.
I listen to the audiobook of *An Enchanted April*, and the

passages that describe the wisteria in bloom and the flower-filled garden bathed in sunlight are a balm. I sleep a great deal, like a melancholic hedgehog.

As the month progresses, the sky clears and the temperature falls. Puddles freeze over, mud hardens so that it thuds as I walk on it, and any remaining woodland fruit is blackened by ice crystals as they pierce and burst the cells of its flesh. This kind of scimitar-sharp winter's day with a pale, low sun in delicate watercolour skies can clear my mind of its stupor. I'm grateful for the invigorating shift in isobars, and my cheeks sting in the iced air as Annie and I tread the familiar paths in the wood. I hear more long-tailed tits in the tops of the young beeches and glimpse them flitting among the dry coppery leaves. We trace the border of the wood from the corner where the hazel grows along the rough hedge of blackthorn that skirts its edge. To our right, beneath the beeches, the whitish chalk-rich soil protrudes in places, and the wild carrot and hedge-parsley seed heads, grasses and a tangle of denuded wild roses make a patchwork of grey and pale brown. Here and there are pools of frost.

Knapweed, a perennial relative of the cornflower, grows here and in June and July forms an intense purple haze of flowers beloved by hoverflies, bees and butterflies. On warm days the flattish, frilly-fringed dark mauve blooms are a good place to observe the state of local insect diversity. Now, in January, their desiccated seed heads that I drew in October still stand.

Wild carrot

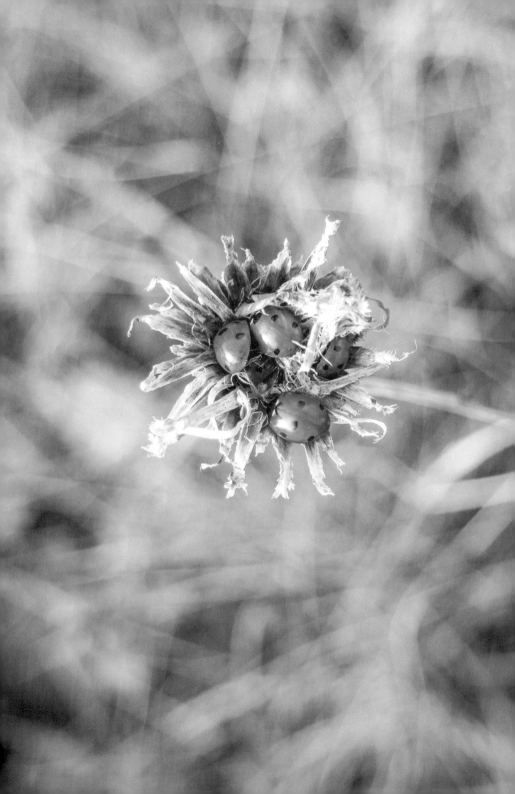

The sun has opened their petal-like scales, forming shapes like miniature dried sunflowers. As I examine them there's a small glimmer of red in my vision and at first I mistake it for a retinal flash caused by bending down too quickly, but it persists and looking more closely I realize that there are ladybirds in the centre of many of the rosettes. In one of them five are nestled, motionless and in the torpor of hibernation. The centres of the seed heads are hairy, trapping air and forming a layer of insulation, preventing frost from penetrating and providing protection for the ladybirds when the temperature drops on clear nights.

There is a reason that ladybirds gather together in groups to overwinter. If a ladybird is attacked by a bird or other predator on a day when it is active it will produce a yellowish fluid from its leg joints called, rather gothically, 'reflex blood'. It is rich in alkaloids and is bitter and foul tasting to birds. Along with its bright coloration, this response is an effective deterrent, and after attempting to eat their first ladybird and receiving a beak full of acrid toxins most birds will avoid them. During winter when their usual aphid or scale-insect food is not available and temperatures drop too low to permit activity, ladybirds must hibernate in order to survive. The production of reflex blood costs energy that the ladybirds do not have to spare and so they no longer produce it in response to an attack between November and March. Instead, the ladybirds huddle together in a place where frost cannot reach them: between the needles of yew, in the curled-up desiccated leaves of beech or in the crook of a branch of wild rose. Should a robin or dunnock decide to chance a wintry ladybird snack, one of the group may be lost but the rest will remain, huddled together and looking at first glance like a rather large insect sporting the warning

‹ Ladybirds hibernating in knapweed seed head

colours of red and black. Most individuals will survive until the days turn warmer in March or April, and their year will begin. The sight of these much-loved beetles couched together in their little vegetal beds brings an exhilaration akin to finding treasure. To me these are beetly rubies. The melancholy that rolled in with the dank weather earlier in the month lifts a little.

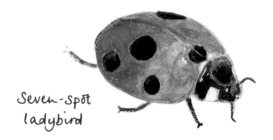

Seven-spot
ladybird

I hear news, news that makes a naturalist's heart leap like Annie when she can smell a sausage. There is a murmuration of starlings, 40,000 strong, soaring and writhing over Walberswick beach each evening, and I see the evidence on Instagram. I know that seeing a huge flock of birds dancing in the air as though they are a single organism will help to banish my wintry gloom, and I long to witness it, so I message my friend Mel, who has just moved to Suffolk. She's a fellow naturalist and is similarly excited at the thought, so I pick her up and we drive to Walberswick, arriving an hour or two before dusk. Crossing a concrete bridge we clamber over the dunes in the direction of Sizewell and an expansive bed of reeds. It seems we share an urge to examine pebbles, and this patch of coastline with its large deposits of sea-worn flint, carnelian, jasper and even Baltic amber means that some of the walk is spent bent over, eyes to the shingle, seeking holed hag stones and rounded egg-like flints.

We walk a high dune path that skirts the reed bed where I have heard that the starlings come to roost. As the light begins to fade and the clouds glow apricot and peach, our eyes are glued to the horizon. 'Ooh, they're coming,' I say excitedly, as a flock of birds emerges from above some distant woodland. As they draw nearer they resolve into rooks, not starlings. Frustratingly, several more corvid flocks pass over, so we distract ourselves by directing our binoculars towards the reeds. A little egret stands sentry at the edge of a pool, then lifts on curved wings. I experience the same thrill at the sight of the egret as I do when I see a grey heron. There is something pterodactyl-like and ancient about the silhouettes of this group of birds. Its movement in the air seems cantilevered and slightly stiff, as though it is a wooden bird mobile and someone has pulled the string attached, launching it into a puppet-like flight.

The sky remains empty of starlings but we refuse to admit defeat. A small tumbling cloud of finches moves across the top of the reeds, but dusk has fallen and neither Mel nor I can tell what they are. The rosy-peach colours of the sky become more vivid and are reflected in the pool where the egret stood. For a few minutes our view is intensely beautiful. We dawdle a while longer, discussing the medicinal properties of soil and our fondness for rooks and watching the colours as they shift. The sky's glow fades, the light becomes grainy, and realizing that the starlings are not coming we walk back along the dunes towards the village. We had no sighting of the writhing mass of birds that we hoped for but a feeling of rightness descends. Time spent on the shore with a friend was restorative and I'm left feeling better for several days afterwards.

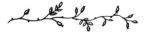

Towards the end of the month I experience a flurry, or rather a parliament, of owl sightings. Like the sparrowhawks in December they seem to coordinate their appearances, as though they have discussed it between themselves and decided that they should show themselves to me in quick succession in the last week of January. One evening, after the children have gone to bed, when anxiety crawls into my mind and spring seems far off, I drive my usual route towards Dullingham, in need of distraction and the soothing feeling of being cocooned in the warm car in the dark.

As I take a left-hand turn towards Haverhill the countryside opens up. Large fields on the left of the road are lined with hogweed seed heads and adolescent sycamores. On the right is a fence edging a field of livestock and as I drive the visual line of the fence seems altered somehow; two dark shapes disturb the rhythm of the palings. I turn at the next farm track and drive back to take a look. My mind leaps as I see two little owls standing like diminutive sentinels on the fence. As the car approaches they take off, making overlapping curved flight paths away from and then back to their posts. Their flight style is slightly frenzied, like that of a puffin or partridge. It has the hint of a bird in a hurry, one that really oughtn't to slow down lest it drop out of the air. It's a comical sight, as are their apparently scowling expressions as they peer at the car. The pattern of feathers on the brow of a little owl is such that it seems to have a permanent glower.

Several days later, I drive to pick up my youngest daughter from the after-school playgroup in the next village. As I pass the row of young lime trees near the local farm shop, a barn owl is sitting on one of the branches, gazing at the grass below. The daylight is almost gone and dusk has descended. The paleness of the bird makes it resemble the photographic negative of a dark owl against a bright sky. Just metres away is a barn in which I know the owls nest. It is part of the farm complex and while visiting the small honesty shop to buy cut flowers in July I had heard a raspy hissing sound coming from the corrugated iron walls of the barn. Beyond the courtyard where I stood I had seen a whirring movement and, walking over to the gate, I caught sight of a barn owl flying into a hole in the wall of the barn just beneath the eaves. The land between the two villages on which the farm sits is a patchwork of fallow fields and native ancient grassland, and the barn owls seem to be thriving here. The barn owl nest was a heartening sign, hinting that there is a healthy population of mice and voles in these fields. Despite the relative frequency with which I see owls here, I never become tired of the sight of them or take it for granted.

The following week I travel to the coast of Suffolk. A tiny converted dairy shed will be home for a few days while I write, take a brief break from parenting and spend a little more time at the coast. My car's headlights scan a neat hedge as I turn a corner in Sibton Green and there, sitting on top of the trimmed privet, is a tawny owl. There are no cars behind me so I stop and the columns of light illuminate the bird, who stands its ground and seems unperturbed. It peers balefully at the car, moving its head from side to side, trying to gather more information about the source of light. Its breast feathers are patterned like oak bark, conferring camouflage and allowing it to sit unnoticed in trees during the day. Patches of pale greyish feathers each side of its beak give it a moustachioed and haughty look.

I have always been in slight awe of tawny owls ever since *The Tale of Squirrel Nutkin* was read to me as a bedtime story when I was a child. The impudent squirrel protagonist taunts and dances about Old Brown the tawny owl, who, pushed beyond the limit of his owly patience, suddenly loses his statue-like composure and pins Nutkin to the ground with his talons. Beatrix Potter's painting of this scene shows Old Brown with a frenzied look, intent on a kill. Nutkin makes a narrow escape, but I always found that painting and the story chilling. It was perhaps the first time that I became aware that nature could be simultaneously bewitching and cruel, and the sight of this tawny atop the hedge reminds me of my childhood dread of Old Brown and that first unnerving sense that the world could be a difficult place.

This owl's feathers look incredibly soft and I find myself longing to touch them. The dense plumage helps to provide warmth, vital for a hunter that often sits and waits for prey rather than actively seeking it. And the outermost flight feathers have a comb-like 'fimbriate margin', which helps disrupt airflow and keep the bird's wingbeats silent as it swoops on its victim. Its expressive forward-facing eyes, which may have lent the notion that owls are wise, are

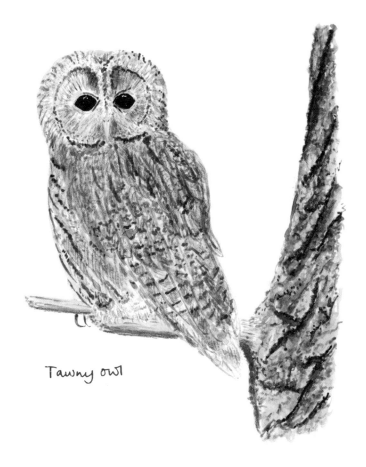

Tawny owl

for gathering as many photons as possible into its retinas, allowing it to see its prey more clearly and ambush it in the owl-light. The characteristics of owls that appeal most to humans are the ones this bird clan have evolved to prey more efficiently on small mammals. My hedge-perching tawny finally decides to move off and lifts away on wings barred with chestnut and chocolate brown.

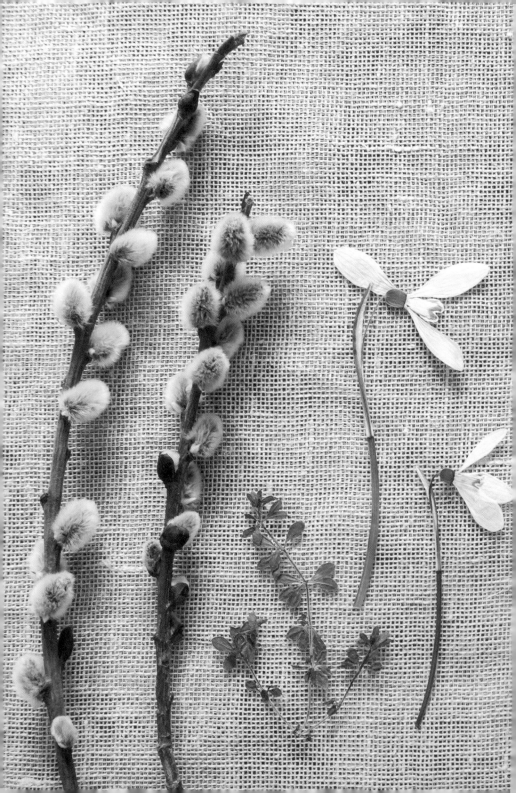

February

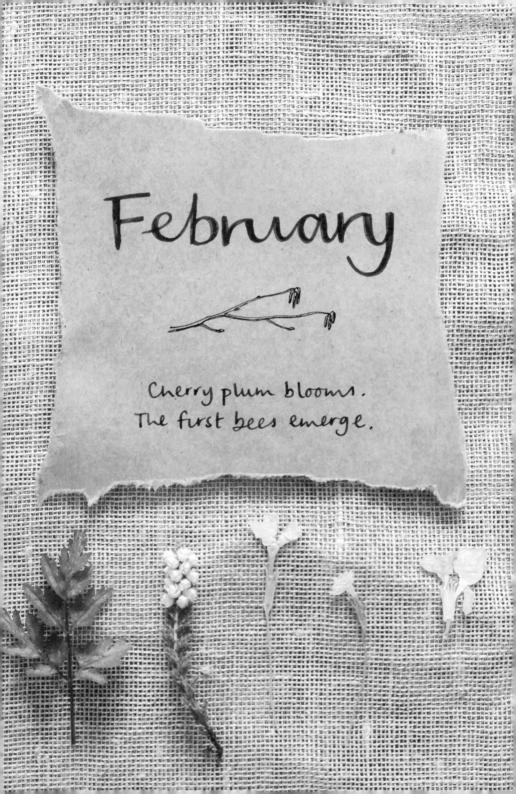

Cherry plum blooms.
The first bees emerge.

The weather since New Year has been colder than that in the same weeks of last year, and the botanical calendar shifts as a result. The molecular clocks within the local flora slow, and the growth of foliage and emergence of flower buds goes into stasis. Since we came to live in this rural Fenland spot, the year has been rendered in my mind as a floral succession, a sort of chronological conveyor belt of flowering plants as the months progress, beginning with aconites and snowdrops in February. This year the familiar relay of wildflowers is slow to begin. Low temperatures have delayed the starting pistol and I itch with impatience. I am determined to seek out as many signs of the changing season as possible.

Snowdrops edge into bud and linger there in suspended animation. Finally, inevitably, they open. Earliest to bloom are the ones in my neighbour's patch of land whose shoots I spotted last month, a giant variety taller than a bluebell with white bells the size of jelly babies. Seeing their flowers as I walk with Annie up to the main wood has such a welcome effect on my brain and I am so glad to see them that I feel almost tearful. Later that week, I see a mass of white beside the road in Exning on my way to the supermarket. Many hundreds of snowdrops are in flower there and it is a good sight – clean and fresh, like the botanical version of new linen. I park the car nearby and photograph them, revelling in their numbers, allowing myself to be reassured by this tangible sign of the changing season.

Snowdrops growing by the side of the road in Exning ›

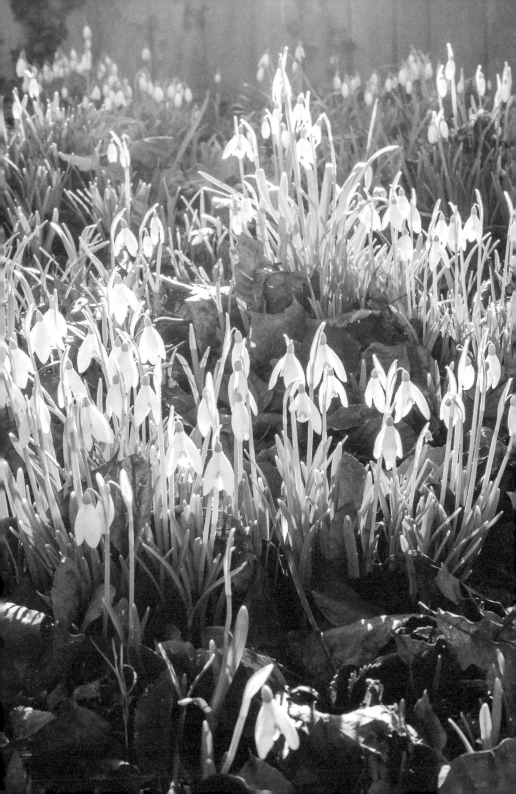

I find the emergence of the first blossom in the vicinity of our cottage to be as uplifting as the arrival of the first swallow. It is confirmation of the approach of spring proper, when the sun warms my back as I walk in the wood, when orange-tip butterflies flit over garlic mustard, and field edges and verges wear intricate lace ruffs of cow parsley. It is a subtle signpost that I find immensely cheering, and I search for it each year with the wide-eyed giddiness of a child on Christmas morning. Wild cherry plum is always first to open its blossom here on the edge of the Fens. It is delicate and ephemeral, with flowers slightly larger than that of blackthorn or wild sloe, marked out by the green slender stems of growth from the previous year.

I drive from Burwell to Exning via a quiet back road where sometimes I see hares in the arable fields. A small patch of established woodland borders the road for several hundred metres, giving way to the characteristic open flat fields and hedges of Fenland. I drive slowly in the hope of seeing a hare, and at the brink of the wood where it gives way to a bridleway and newly ploughed soil there is a muted glimmer, a little extra light. Perhaps it was litter trapped among the branches, perhaps scraps of late winter sky visible through the hedge. I pull over. There it is, the first blossom of the year. Tiny delicate white floral cups garland a very few branches of cherry plum.

In China and Japan early plum blossom, *meihua* (Chinese) or *ume* (Japanese), is revered due to its appearance when the land is still in the grip of winter and because it can bloom when snow still covers the ground. Yet it is also a sign of impending spring, so it is simultaneously a symbol of two seasons as they intersect. So significant are these flowers that *ume* is depicted in literature and ancient paintings, and is even rendered in rice paste to form special sweets, while the Japanese word for plum is used as a *kigo* (a word or phrase associated with a particular season) for spring in *haiku* and *renga* poetic verses. Early plum blossom is purported to be a talisman against evil and is often planted in the northeast of Japanese gardens, the direction from which dark forces are supposed to emanate. This English cherry plum, a cousin of the Asian versions that are feted, painted and mused upon, has far smaller flowers, and I wonder whether anyone has noticed it here, heralding warmer days in a very tiny way along the hem of a stark Fenland field. When I return to the house I mark this small but important sighting with a pencil drawing.

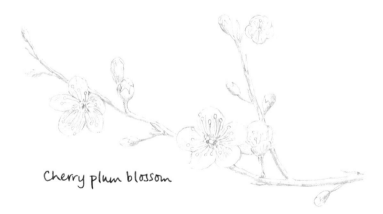

Cherry plum blossom

Storm clouds of difficult thoughts rumble at the edges of my consciousness; my brain needs the solace of landscape and I set out on what I hope will be a curative drive. During such car journeys I often keep the windows open, even in winter, as the cold air enlivens my senses and can rouse me from gloom. Beyond Dullingham I take a new route. The roads are winding, tall hedges form corridors along the way and when the scenery opens before me there is a muted palette of greys, browns and tired winter greens, like a quilt sewn from utility fabrics, rather rough and worn. There is little in these views that lifts my spirits but it is better than skulking in our north-facing cottage and yearning for spring.

There is an hour or so until dusk and, as I drive, the cloud cover begins to disperse, revealing a delicate lucent sky the colour of a starling's egg. As the sun edges towards the horizon, shafts of winter light seem to emanate from the tops of the hedgerows as I pass. I continue for some time, enjoying the gentle roll of the countryside as I move further into Suffolk. I drive along the main road through Carlton Green, passing a jumble of seventeenth- and eighteenth-century pastel-painted cottages, until I reach the centre of the village where, next to a signpost marking a crossroads, I find a beautiful sight: a stand of artichoke seed heads, as tall as I am, silhouetted against the winter sky. Each stem ends in a fiercely spiked sphere that makes me think of medieval weapons. The huge toothed thistle-like leaves curve downwards to touch the surrounding sward like the wings of a swan. This is not a wild sight; someone planted these artichokes here, but their statuesque proportions, the dramatic shapes they make against the sky and their backdrop of undulating farmland and woodland elicits that familiar exhilaration that can be caused by a tiny speedwell, a filigree of frost on a fallen leaf or the sight of a fulmar tucked into its nest on Hunstanton cliffs. Just now this feeling is especially welcome and I stop the car and stand gazing at the artichokes. I photograph them to remind myself of this sight, so that I can look back at it during the remaining days of winter – days that I know will be the most difficult.

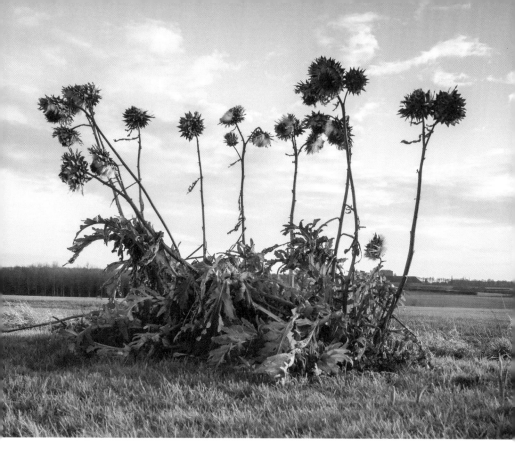

^ Artichoke seed heads at Carlton Green, Suffolk

I continue along this new route as the sun sinks yet lower. Furthest from its glow there is a vivid blue; a line drawn from this point along the meridian towards the sunset would traverse the subtlest ombre, from deep indigo to the colour of peach flesh. There is no cloud and every branch, leaf and fence paling shows dark and crisp against the blues and golds. Stands of teasels line the right-hand verge. In one place there are hundreds, perhaps thousands of them. Silhouetted *en masse* they look like a crowd of Giacometti's elongated and rather unnerving sculptures of human figures. Teasel seeds are a favourite food for goldfinches during winter; this mass of seed heads is like a giant supermarket for them and I wonder whether charms of goldfinches gather here during the day. I resolve to return to find out.

I turn a corner and catch sight of a barn owl flying slowly over the verge to my left. I pull over to watch it. It hovers for a few moments and drops down into the long grass. I wait, captivated by what I have just witnessed. After some moments, I realize that I'm holding my breath, and then the owl lifts from the grass. I am parked just a few metres from it. The bird ignores the car, flies low over the road and alights in a field on the other side of the carriageway. As it passes I see a small grey body and a short tail in its talons: a vole. I turn the car around and drive to a large lay-by near the place where the owl descended into the field. There it is, sitting on the grass part, hidden behind the

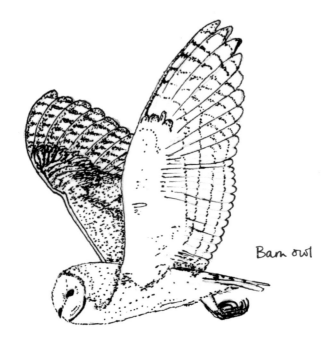

Barn owl

hedge, shoulders hunched. I presume it is having its meal and has chosen this spot because it is sheltered. The sun has almost reached the horizon as the owl continues to eat, and the trees and hedgerows become haloed with gold. It is one of the most beautiful sights I have witnessed in nature. It reminds me that however exhausted I am by depression, however often it tricks my thoughts, leadens my limbs and bleakens my outlook, it is worth striving to suffuse my brain with medicinal elation from encounters like this.

No other human saw the owl hunting in these few square metres of Suffolk or saw it in the field having its meal. The owl took just seconds to make its kill, and shortly after it dropped down behind the hedge to feed, it lifted away on its pale wings. It was so brief, yet I feel immensely privileged to have witnessed it. I know that barn owls live and breed just half a mile from my house; they must catch food every day, but I have seen this owl hunting successfully right in front of me and it is like the moment in Pembrokeshire in the early 1980s when I saw barnacles open tiny trapdoors and begin to feed in the seawater I had collected in my bucket.

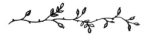

Each week that brings the calendar closer to March there is a shift in the position of the northern hemisphere in relation to the sun. We gain a little more sunlight every day, the mean temperature rises a fraction of a degree, the enzymes within plants become more active and in many species cells begin to divide. The growing season is beginning. As February progresses beech buds swell, primroses begin to open, the leaves of the cow parsley seedlings that I have found so encouraging in the last four months expand and new embryonic growth appears. Blackthorn branches develop tiny clusters of blossom buds, each one barely bigger than a pinhead. I stop to examine them as Annie and I trudge our familiar routes through the wood, and there is a muted cloud of joy – muted because I haven't finished scaling winter. Spring proper is still not yet here.

However, I know that one of the botanical signposts marking the shift from winter to spring may be about to emerge. Finding evidence of it will be significant for me: it is concrete proof of the shifting of the season and of tree sap beginning to move. This natural sight, although subtle, is very important for local bees. Goat willow and grey willow flowers provide one of the earliest prolific sources of pollen for bumble-bee queens as they search for new places to establish a colony, or for solitary bees, who must build up their energy levels in order to mate and lay eggs in April or May. Both species have the colloquial name pussy willow, as the male flowers, which can emerge as early as February, are covered in fine grey hairs and have a feline silkiness beloved by children.

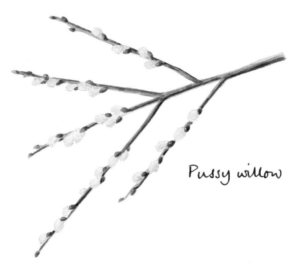

Pussy willow

I wrap myself in coat, shawl, mittens and boots, and walk out of the village onto the edge of the Fen. Beyond a large corrugated iron barn where fodder is stored is a hedgerow full of hawthorn, blackthorn, sycamore, field maple, and the particular trees I am seeking. I have almost reached Tubney Fen before I see the first pussy willow of the year. A very few flowers have begun to emerge from the shiny brown bud cases. I touch one with the tip of my finger: the hairs of the flower are so soft that it almost feels as though my skin is touching air. There is a strong biting wind and an unforgiving drizzle driving sideways onto my face, but here it is. I am surrounded by grey, brown, faded green, and the cold is boring into me, but this is as cheering a sight to me as a full roast dinner with extra Yorkshire puddings.

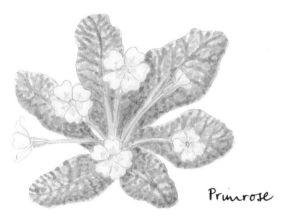

Primrose

It's happened: the end of winter is approaching and the earliest signs of spring proper are evident in wood and hedgerow. During the past four months, when seasonal depression has clawed at my thoughts like so many persistent leg-dragging, moaning zombies among my neurons, I have managed to lift away from it by spending time among trees, plants and wildlife. I have been to the coast, visited water-, wood- and grassland, and dosed myself up with the sight of strutting starlings and the vivid green of new cleavers seedlings. I've walked in all weathers, each trudge shifting the dial of my brain chemistry a little and helping me to persevere. Sometimes the seemingly simple tasks of getting washed, dressed, booted and out of the house in order to drive away despondency have been like scaling a mountain, but most days I've managed the foothills at least, enough to continue to work, to write and, most importantly, to parent.

Keeping depression at bay requires constant vigilance; it's a daily battle requiring the benign artillery of nature walks, time spent creatively if possible and, when I'm alone in the house, the company of a hairy amber-coloured four-legged pal. When workloads are greater than usual, family stresses build up and viruses lurk, the balance can shift. The beneficial effects of being outdoors can be diminished, or rather, the inexorable downward trawl of the depression is stronger. At such times this incessant, exhausting disease can begin to triumph. I'm weary from fighting it and my energy reserves are running very low. I'm longing for warmer days and for the Fenland sunshine to gather strength. As February ends and more wild cherry plum blossom appears, I turn down offers of work and I sleep more; my urge to draw, to collect and to photograph my nature finds ebbs away. I begin to feel detached from all that I'm doing. I fear my depression may be gaining ground.

Teasels and sunset near Carlton Green, Suffolk >

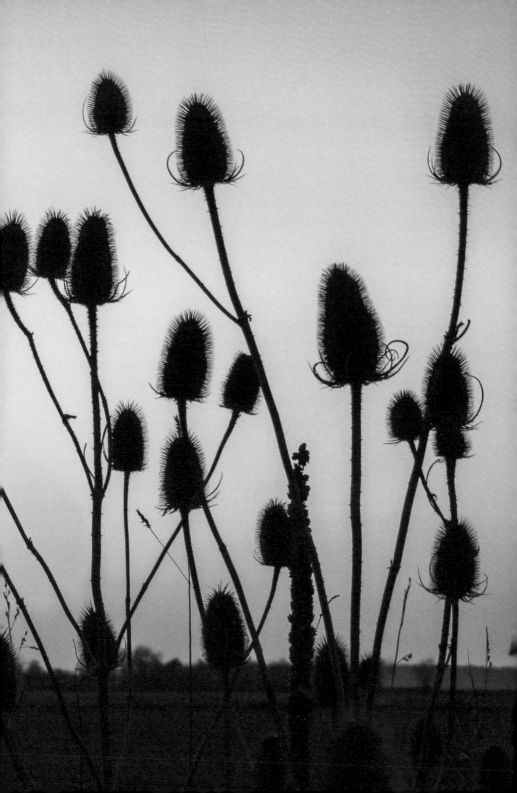

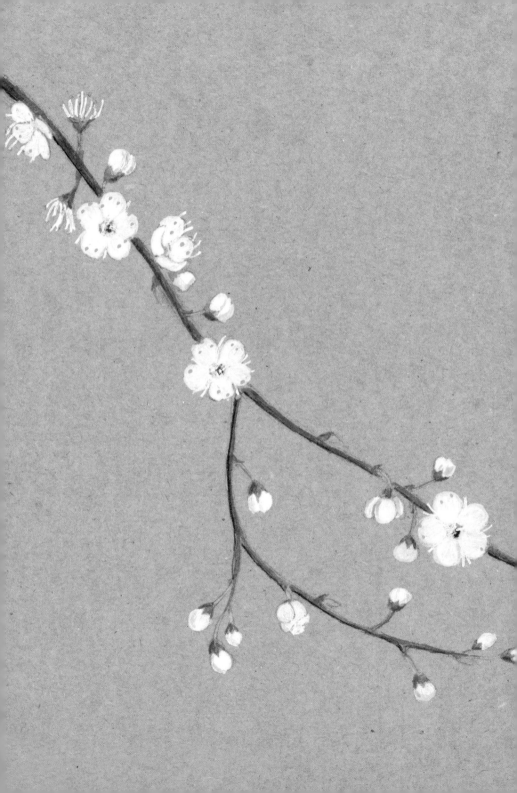

March

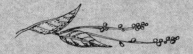

Hawthorn leaves emerge.
Blackthorn blooms.

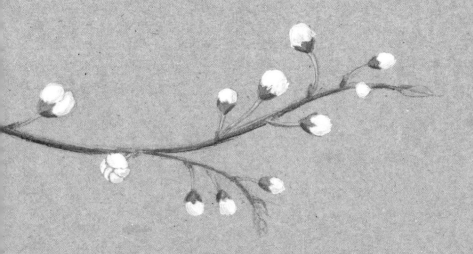

At the beginning of March I return to Suffolk, determined to witness the murmuration that Mel and I sought in January. I see on Twitter that another flock of around 40,000 starlings is appearing at Minsmere and roosting in the brambles and reeds there. When I arrive at the reserve there is less than an hour until dusk, a persistent drizzle is falling and the light levels are low: an unpromising prospect. I make my way through the visitor centre and out onto the paths that lead across the reserve towards the shore. The rain has become heavier, but at the far end of a path that skirts the reed beds a small group of people are gathered, hoods up, cameras ready. I realize they must have come to see the starlings. I join them and ask if the murmuration has been spotted yet. Rather gloomy faces peep out from beneath hoods. Heads are shaken. 'They don't come every night. They may not come at all.'

We stand damply in the grey light, looking hopefully inland. Someone calls out, 'They're coming!' but it is a flock of pigeons, a false alarm. Several more minutes pass. Suspense and hope hang between us. Then a small indistinct shape, slightly darker than the raincloud behind it, appears above distant woodland. It approaches the shore, and elsewhere in the sky a hazy ribbon of grey appears, snaking as it moves towards the reed bed. '*This* is it. Now they are here,' says the woman standing next to me. More small flocks advance, flying well above tree height, each of them writhing in the sky. Suddenly the air is full of starlings flying directly overhead, and we crane our necks to watch them. When they fly close to us I feel as though I am among them, soaring and swarming with thousands of companions. It gives me a heady, vertiginous sensation, similar to the times when I lived in London in my twenties,

had drunk rather too much wine, took the tube home and
closed my eyes. The train seemed to fly upwards and defy
gravity. Surrounded by these tumbling, twirling birds, I feel
similarly giddy.

As I watch the changing shapes and movements of
the flocks, my mind is filled with imagery. A large group
flies out to sea, then swerves, making a speckled arc, like
interference on an untuned television, as the birds shift
direction and move back inland. These starlings, thousands
of them now, are behaving like drops of mercury shaken on
a saucer: small groups gather, split apart, then fuse again. In
some parts of the sky they mass closely, like swarms of bees;
in others, snaking strands of birds squirm above the trees.

Then we spy a dark silhouette. A larger bird is there
at the outskirts of one of the flocks. I presume it is a
sparrowhawk, but a closer look through binoculars reveals
sickle-shaped wings as it banks in the sky. Is it? I think it is:
a peregrine falcon. I have only seen a peregrine once before,
on a student field trip in 1991, it was flying over the cliffs
on Skomer Island while choughs strutted below and puffins
floated in rafts on the waves. This bird is nearer now and it
is hunting. Research from the University of Bristol shows
that murmurations are larger and more dense if raptors are
hunting among the starlings. It is thought that this helps to
confuse the predators. The peregrine's presence is a threat
to the birds and has induced them to make an even more
impressive and complex display.

The murmuration itself is a wonder, a sight that inspires
awe, but seeing a peregrine among them seeking a meal
has a more marked effect on me. Having spent so much of
winter pinned in by heavy thoughts, barely able to move
mentally or physically, these few minutes witnessing such

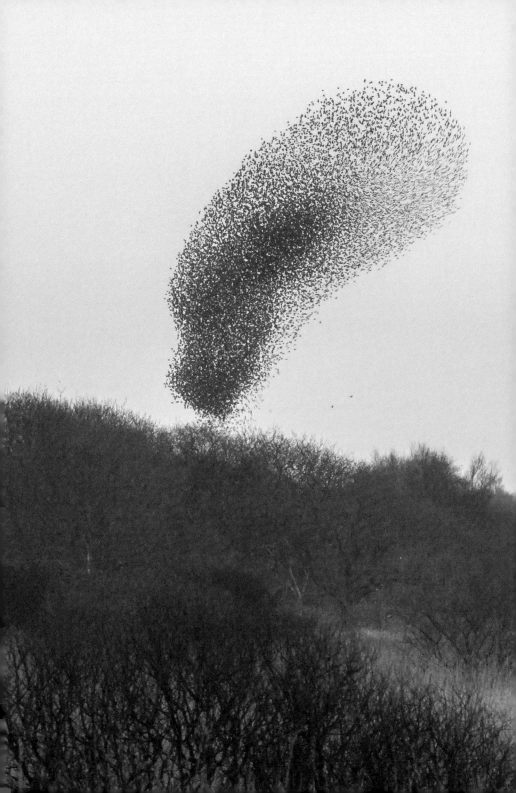

an enormous and wild spectacle, a bird of prey hawking among tens of thousands of dancing starlings, is setting my mind apart from the blackness and providing respite.

The preliminary dance seems to be over because now, on some signal known by all the starlings, the separate groups begin to converge to make one gargantuan, pulsating form. The smaller flocks enter the main group by plummeting en masse: they drop suddenly into the core of the murmuration, each flock an ornithological waterfall swelling the numbers of their companions below. Tens of thousands of birds are behaving like a living liquid. My mind reels at the complexity of the mathematics and silent communication required for this astonishing behaviour.

Now the murmuration is huge. Writhing limbs of birds, coordinated by their brains' responses to one another's flightpaths, protrude then recede from its edge as it seems to crawl like an aerial amoeba. One moment it echoes the molten draping shape of a Dali clock, then a spiralling millipede, and all the while the 40,000 move as one. As the birds shift so that their bodies are silhouetted against the rainclouds, a dark wave moves across the flock. When these densely black furrows of birds travel through the murmuration, a bubble of quiet exhilaration suffuses my brain. It is poorly articulated and muffled, but some joy is there. I know that if I were able to watch this, one of nature's most humbling spectacles, in late summer or early autumn, my response would be more potent, that it would penetrate more deeply into my conscious and subconscious mind. Since November a pall of despondency has grown, become thick and opaque in my neurons, and formed a resistant barrier to positive experiences. Yet in these moments, in the presence of the starlings' implausibly

< Starling murmuration at RSPB Minsmere

beautiful dance, I do enjoy a separation from the darkness. It is over now, though. The sky has lost all light and the starlings have roosted. I am left feeling thoughtful and grateful and yet rather numb. I am glad I persisted in seeking it out and I know this will be one of the most incredible things I will ever see, but its effects do not last.

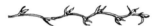

Despite the wonder of the murmuration the last vestiges of mental energy that had been sustaining me throughout winter ebb away when I return home. The lack of sunlight and the incessant daily effort needed to defy this illness in the last five months has taken its toll. My brain chemistry shifts significantly and I plummet, sinking through the flimsy floor of positive thought and down the precipitous frictionless walls of depression's deepest well. The cherry plum blossom has opened and is followed by blackthorn, but I am unaware of these signs of spring. The changes in local nature that I have so longed for since October are beginning to take place, but my focus is now on trying to gain some traction, any small foothold, against the well's sheer walls.

The mental effort required to move my body becomes overwhelming. My daily to-do lists change from January's 'finish article, photograph primroses, pitch piece' to March's 'have bath, eat breakfast, brush teeth'. These small tasks are all I can manage. Some days I cannot tick anything off my list. The shift in my brain chemistry weighs me down and it becomes difficult to move.

Enjoyment drains away from all things like water through the Dungeness shingle. Even fried foods lose their allure; even cheese. Cheese, my dear fermented salty

umami-laden friend, no longer induces that all-enveloping
satisfaction of intense savouriness. It tastes of nothing;
of paste and emptiness. I eat very sharp salt and vinegar
crisps and acerbic satsumas, trying to awaken the part of
my brain that, when I'm well, lights up with a cocktail
of neurotransmitters and electrical signals whenever I eat
something delicious. Now the response to these sharp
flavours is muted, deadened, the joy of eating gone. My
collection of beautiful soft yarns feels like hessian, straw,
and my usual urge to loop them into mittens and shawls,
relishing the silken fibres, the smoothness of the crochet
hook and the patterns made by the strands as my hands
make the stitches, evaporates. When this disease eats
my mind like an insatiable grey slug, it feels as though
the responses of my entire body and every sense become
dormant. My brain's pleasure centres are not functioning
properly and this induces more melancholy. I miss the
deliciousness of a freshly fried chip and the unctuous high
of chocolate cake. Losing pleasure in this way is called
anhedonia and is a common symptom of depression. The
illness seems cunning, calculating in this deprivation. It is
cannibalistic, feeding on itself, and as it steals pleasure so it
strengthens its grip on the brain.

The causes of depression are still relatively poorly
understood. Serotonin-processing pathways are depleted
in depressed and suicidal patients, so drugs such as SSRIs
(selective serotonin reuptake inhibitors) that raise levels
of serotonin are used to treat it. This group of drugs is
effective for many patients, but for a third of depressed
people they have little or no effect, which suggests that
other biochemical changes take place in a depressed
brain. For example, levels of norepinephrine, another

neurotransmitter, are also altered during prolonged periods of low mood and are boosted by some SSRIs. There are undoubtedly more biochemical changes linked to depression that are yet to be discovered. Chronic stress is a common factor in many cases, leading to raised levels of the stress hormone cortisol, and if sources of stress continue to be present for long periods, the risk of depression is higher. New research is beginning to show that there may even be a link between gut flora, the cortisol pathway and depression. These changes in hormonal, neurochemical and biome systems are clues to the mechanism of this illness, but it is a highly complex condition and more research is needed to understand these connections in much more detail.

My world narrows. I stay in the cottage and move slowly between its rooms. My thoughts become sluggish and jumbled and ideas for drawings, photographs and writing vanish. I avoid friends and turn down invitations to socialize. I can manage only the simplest tasks each day, and the guilt I feel about my inability to contribute to the household, fulfil work commitments and be an engaged parent is overwhelming. Self-reproach brings my mind lower still.

At first I try to continue. I work from bed as best I can; I continue to write during the short periods when my mind is more alert. Sleep dominates everything: I can barely stay awake and have three, sometimes four naps a day along with a full night's sleep. My memory blurs, and several times I find that the end of the day has arrived and I was barely aware that it had begun.

There are compartments in my brain in which I keep the most difficult things that have happened: the consequences of a grandparent's death when I was nineteen;

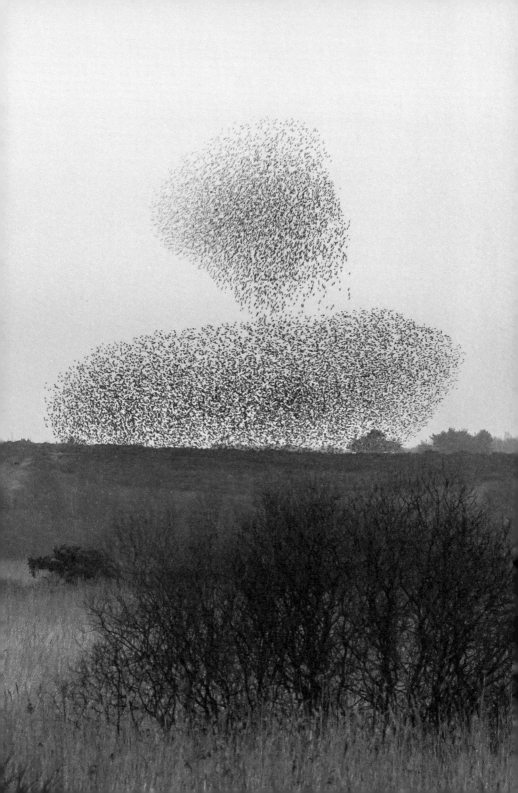

the second university degree I was too ill to complete; a very unsettled, seemingly unhappy baby, the impact it had on my confidence as a mother and the resultant loss of a friendship; the severe brain injury of a family member and the coldness and rejection of neighbours when I spoke about it; certain family relationships that are disjointed and may never be functional.

Each item in this list is represented here by a very few words, yet each is as complex and painful as a stand of steel brambles tangled among my frontal lobes. I have addressed each as best I can with talking cures and the pharmaceutical balm of antidepressants. I have mustered as much acceptance as I am able and then nailed each into a box in my mind as tightly as I can manage. The baby was unsettled because she responded to the world in a slightly different way. I wasn't doing anything wrong, although at the time I was entirely convinced that I was, and as a result my post-natal depression was severe. The brain injury was a terrible accident that altered a life and the lives around it. The neighbours simply did not want to contemplate a damaged, non-functioning brain. It made them think of death, so they recoiled from me when I spoke of it. At the time I felt like an outcast: they excluded me from social contact that had been a lifeline, and I struggled to understand why they were behaving in such a way. But perhaps those were not the best people to be among at that time.

I am reconciled to many of these things now and no longer blame myself, but in the sides of the boxes in which I have stowed these jagged, piercingly painful happenings are invisible gaps, imperceptible holes through which memories seep and colour my outlook on life. The effects of winter's dearth of light is overlaid on these memories, and when

combined with the chronically high level of adrenaline and
cortisol caused by certain aspects of our family life it can
be difficult to extricate my mind from the thorny tangle.
The lack of sunlight in winter shifts my brain chemistry
and dampens my mood for a month or two either side of
Christmas. Now, in March, I'm dragged downwards, all
the boxes seem to fly open and an overpowering self-hatred
and self-chastisement that is not logical, is not needed, yet
will not be quietened, erupts in my mind. This is the most
dangerous weapon in depression's armoury. Ironically, early
spring, despite its promise of sunlight and growth, is often the
most difficult time for me to keep the lowest, most sinister
mental state at bay. My thoughts swirl and my mind is swept
into a maelstrom made up of scathing self-recriminations that
endlessly list the ways in which I didn't do things properly,
do not manage anything well enough, am clearly a piece of
shit. Fractured memories of the things I haven't managed
to achieve, and of others' coldness and criticism, fuel my
thoughts: they behaved like that because there is something
wrong with me; I didn't do things right; I am no good. The
storm is insatiable and as it churns it seeks out evidence for
its sole assertion: that I am worth nothing. The din becomes
unbearably loud and takes over my mind completely.

Suicidal ideation is a rather benign-sounding medical
term for what begins to manifest itself in my thoughts in
mid-March. This is the black hole of depression: an event
horizon at which gravity is terrifyingly strong. Exhausted
by the winter and the chemical alteration it inflicts on my
brain, by incessant unavoidable stresses and by unrealistic
self-inflicted pressures, my resistance to the inexorable pull
of depression's ultimate goal fizzles to nothing. My mind
lurches towards the self-ablation that this illness craves.

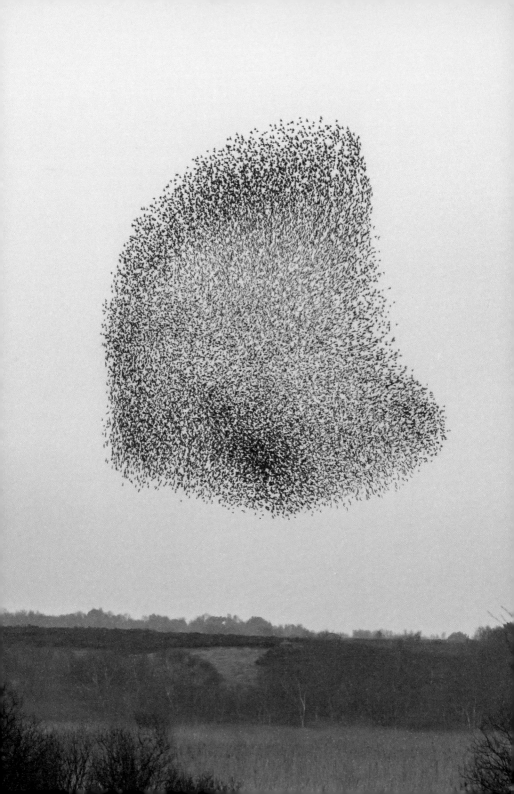

I think of ways in which I could do it. The thoughts are
so powerful that the distraction techniques I am able to
employ for most days of the year to keep well away from
this precipice are nowhere. It feels as though I am poised at
the top of the Niagara Falls in a tiny dinghy.

I drive to the A11. There are bridges there. My
thoughts are loud and incessant, focused on this research.
Which bridge would be best? Most effective? Highest?
The cacophony is terrifying. It feels physical, as though
my mind is actually bursting from my skull. The urge to
end myself roars in my mind. As I drive I catch sight of
the scrubby saplings growing in the central reservation.
The glimpses of green and the hum and rhythm of the car
quieten the cannibalistic clamour. A part of my brain that
has been silent for days awakens: the part that is my own
well self, the part which seeks out nature as a remedy. 'You
are not well,' it says; 'seek help.' The voice is very, very
small, but I listen. I continue along the A11 for some time,
allowing the car to soothe my mind a little more. I pass
more trees. Trees: green, relief. My mind is not still, but
the terrible churning and lurching towards that point of
no return has ceased. There is some quiet. I drive home. I
tell my husband how unwell I am. I go to bed and distract
myself with films: scenes of the past, bustled frocks, neatly
concluded stories, escapism. He brings me cups of tea and
good food. The following morning I go to the doctor and a
recovery plan is made: rest, a higher dose of antidepressants,
appointments to speak with a mental health support team.
The doctor gives me the number of a place I can stay if my
dark notions become overwhelming. So begins the slow
difficult crawl away from that place where my thoughts
wanted me gone.

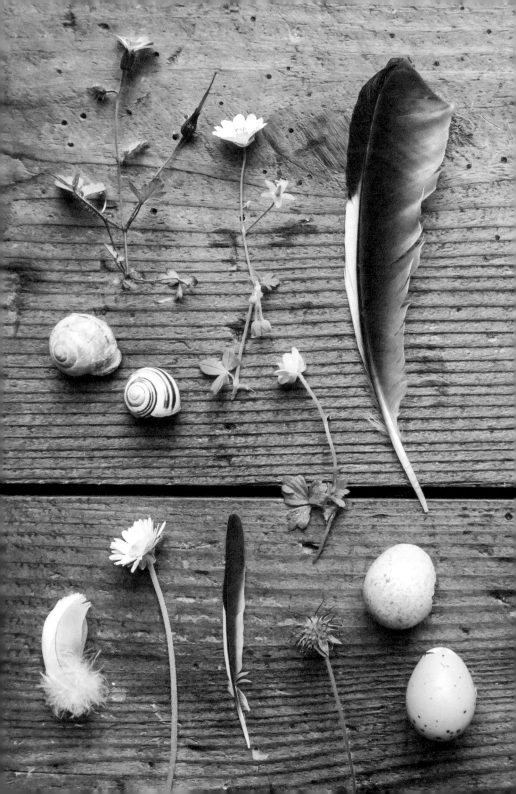

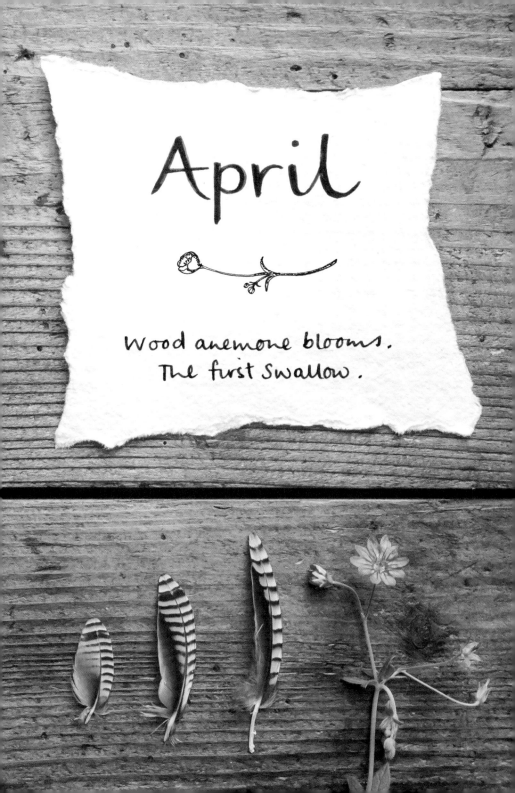

April

Wood anemone blooms.
The first swallow.

Anyone might be forgiven for taking a look at my situation and questioning why I suffer from depression at all: a bonny cottage, a marriage, two children, a small business that's doing okay. These are all very, very good things, and I am hugely grateful for them, but this illness doesn't care who you are or how you live. Admittedly, daily life is tough for my family. There is a great deal of stress and exhaustion, and sometimes it feels as though we are firefighting constantly just to keep going. A line-up of difficult events – accidents, severe illnesses, their aftermath and other peoples' reactions to these things – happened in quick succession over the course of three years or so and changed our situation drastically. As each tricky circumstance occurred, the black dog rubbed its paws gleefully, packed its bags and ultimately moved in to my frontal lobes on a permanent basis in 2008. Sometimes, when I'm especially exhausted, it has a massive party and invites over its pals Crippling Anxiety and Suicidal Ideation for a knees-up. This is what happened last month.

The particular neuronal state that occurred in my brain in March can be fatal. I find it helpful to look this fact in the eye on days when I chastise myself for showing symptoms of depression. A suicidal state of mind feels significantly different to that experienced on an average depressive day. Thoughts are faster, rather like running down a steep hill, and they seem to be spurred on by a loud and urgent need to self-obliterate. In fact, there is some evidence that suicidal brains are different. A neurotransmitter called gamma amino

butyric acid (GABA) acts as a kind
of dampener to neuronal activity.
In the brains of suicide victims
one of GABA's receptors is
expressed at lower levels, meaning
that its moderating effects are reduced. This
would fit with the racing, tumbling, negative
thoughts I had in March. They ran riot and
it was a struggle to find ways to silence them
and their sinister intentions. It is thought that
this change in suicidal brains is epigenetic. That is,
the shift in GABA receptor expression and activity
is caused by our environment influencing the way in
which our genes are expressed, which in turn influences
our neuronal activity. Which in essence means that
suicidal thoughts might be caused by a series of difficult
circumstances or life events. This GABA-focused research
hints at the mechanisms that lead to the most severe cases
of depression, but in truth the exact biochemical causes of
suicidal thoughts are poorly understood.

As I am writing this several months later, my mind is
different. I cannot say that I feel sated with joy but I'm
all right. I'm looking after my daughter, who has a mild
stomach virus. I have given her a gentle creative task and
she's content. I'm working: painting a wren and writing.
I have eaten and so has she. The washing machine is
making reassuring whirring sounds as its cycle progresses.
I can hear a male blackbird singing in our garden hedge,
telling the neighbouring birds that this place, our garden,
is his territory. The blackbird gives me a burst of ... yes,
happiness. It is a lyrical, ephemeral, nostalgic sound that
causes bright flashes of colour in my mind. Things are

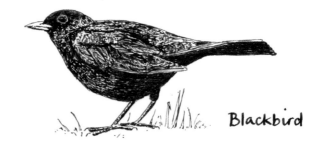

Blackbird

okay. The state of darkness that I described last month is not present as I write now and the relief is enormous, but I have been immersed in it several times during my life, and it is as sinister and lethal as an obsidian knife.

As April begins, my depression lifts a very little but the tempest that took place in my brain in March is still rumbling. While it was at its peak it felt like every nerve ending in my frontal lobes was burning fiercely. At the time I was surprised that it made no sound, as in my head it seemed to roar like constant neuronal thunder that I longed to be able to quieten. The experience was like trying to tend to six screaming vomiting babies simultaneously while someone whispered unconscionably awful things in my ear.

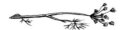

After I visit the doctor I spend much of my time sleeping. The increased dose of SSRI antidepressant has an immediate deadening, sedating effect on my mind, and, besides, I'm tired. In the aftermath of this depressive episode it feels as though my nerve endings are charred from the fierce silent burning: as though my brain circuits have fused and there is a kind of shutdown that takes place afterwards. I know distraction of any kind will help me, but my energy levels have diminished to tiny glimmers: getting out for walks when I'm in recovery can be almost impossible. Films help, and binge-watching the fabulous sequin-encrusted strutting on *RuPaul's Drag Race* keeps me going during much of April. My ability to appreciate soft, beautiful yarns returns in a small way, and as recent building work on our cottage has resulted in long periods without heating I crochet some fingerless mittens for my youngest daughter. Making the stitches is soothing and repetitive, and I feel a small sense of achievement when I see her wearing them. I go to stay with my friend Charlotte to escape the immense guilt of not being able to help a great deal with my family and with keeping the household going. The change of environment helps for a day or two, but my mind dips again and I return home. Besides, I do not want to show Charlotte the depths of inanimate despair that occur when I am at my lowest. The sinking blackness is still present.

I read about research conducted by the University of Exeter that shows how the presence of birds in a landscape can help to lift depression. I decide to attempt some ornithological self-medication and try to encourage birds into our garden. In previous bouts of this illness I have noticed that having a small project to focus on can help to lift my mind away from unbearable self-feeding guilt and sadness. The making of the mittens was an example of this and I am keen to find another. I treat myself to a beautiful handmade wrought-iron feeding station

April

that looks like a slender tree with gnarled branches. With a little energy conferred by the possibility of watching blue tits through the window, I take my daughters to the local garden centre and we fill our basket with bird snacks: mealworms, peanuts, niger seed, fat balls, a sort of muesli for robins and several feeders. We return home, erect the tree-like station near the window and fill the feeders. We have not hung out food for birds for several years, so I have low expectations. I hope that a few feathered visitors might arrive in a week or so, but within twenty-four hours a blue tit begins feeding enthusiastically, followed quickly by a house sparrow.

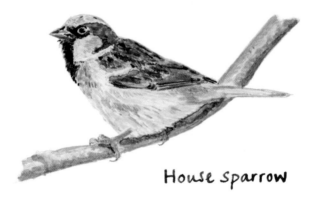

House sparrow

In the days that follow, a gaggle of sparrows become regular visitors, along with a great tit, a pair of goldfinches, a starling and, to my utter delight, a small flock of long-tailed tits. I adore these little birds. They are tiny and charismatic, like energetic feathered lollipops, and their colloquial names include 'bumbarrel', due to their almost spherical nests, and 'flying teaspoon'. It's thrilling to hear the same high-pitched communication calls in our

own garden as I heard in the woods the day I saw them
making their looping flights among the winter branches
in December. When I venture into the garden they don't
seem frightened by my presence, and they stay and feed,
chattering to one another and flitting in and out of the
hedge as they take their turns at the feeders. I sit wrapped
in a huge cardigan and scarf against the spring cold while
I watch them. A glow of gratitude towards these tiny birds
erupts and I can feel a change in mind. This is medicinal.
It's like a live bird channel in the back garden and it's
helping to banish the gloom.

As I sit with a cup of tea one morning after our girls
have left for school, there is a commotion of wings, a blur
of pink-black-white-blue, and a jay lands on the ground
next to the feeding station. I have never seen a jay in the
garden before, but the outdoor bird restaurant we've created
is worthy of a Michelin star, so I suppose it has begun to
attract more unusual diners. The jay cocks its head on one
side to eye the mealworms in the feeder above. Meanwhile
there is a flurry nearby. The male blackbird who has a nest
in our garden hedge becomes incandescent with bird rage
at the sight of the jay. He scampers up to it and starts to
shout with loud, sharp tweets. With each sound he makes
his wings flex to the side, like a person delivering an angry
tirade and waving their arms for emphasis. The blackbird
seems livid and with good reason. Jays are corvids, members
of the crow family, and often raid the nests of other birds
for eggs, nestlings and fledglings. In fact, the jay is seeking
the peanuts and mealworms, but the blackbird cannot risk
losing his brood. Despite being significantly smaller, he
flings himself towards the jay in a frenzy, making to peck it.
Meanwhile, I hear Annie whining as she watches this bird

drama unfold through the window. The jay hops sideways to avoid the blackbird and pecks calmly at a mealworm on the ground. The blackbird seems to consider his position, then retreats to the hedge with a loud, tumbling, angry alarum and continues to spink and tweet at the jay from a distance.

Among my nature collections I have three small precious jay feathers that are hatched with black and the vivid blue of a clear July sky. Such feathers are tricky to find and are sometimes traded and swapped among naturalists as they are so highly prized. I take these three feathers out and gaze at them while the jay is in the garden. They have come from a small patch of colour on the bird's wing. I wonder whether jay feathers were perhaps traded like currency in the past. I'd more than happily swap a side of bacon or a couple of massive cakes for a jay feather or two. To me, they're like bona fide treasure. Despite the hunting prowess of these birds, they are rather timid, so the sight of this one in our garden being dressed down by a snarky blackbird delivers a modest dose of nature-induced antidepressant that I haven't experienced for many weeks. The next day the jay is joined by its mate and I'm thrilled.

The mental energy needed for a walk in the woods still eludes me most days, so I take to sitting by the window and watching the feathered traffic at the feeder. This seemingly insignificant and arguably artificially generated contact with nature keeps me going through many dark days in April.

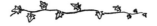

While I was ill last month the spring's progress was once again halted for several weeks by perishingly cold temperatures, snow and harsh frosts. I barely noticed

it happen. I simply observed it detachedly through the
bedroom window, saw charming wintry landscapes and
unfeasibly tall piles of snow atop garden tables appear on
Twitter and Instagram, and eventually became rather bored
of it. At the time, my mind was gripped by a different
kind of winter, and I didn't consider the impact this severe
weather had on wildlife. Not only did the cold snap halt
the gradual increase in both soil and air temperatures that
permit plants and trees to come into leaf and blossom, but
the snow obscured, or locked away in an icebox, ground-
based food such as worms, seeds and small mammals. As a
result, the condition of both male and female birds of many
species deteriorated. A great deal of energy is required to
claim a territory, seek out a mate, build a nest, lay eggs and
then incubate and raise a brood. When wintry weather hits
just as spring begins, it can have a catastrophic effect on the
timing of the pairing-up of many birds. Females must wait
to breed until they are back in condition, and this delay
might prevent pairs from rearing an extra brood during the
breeding season.

Blackbirds have built a nest in our hedge every year for
the past five years. It's a dense garden border of privet, elder
and box. I am not sure whether it is the same blackbird
pair building the nest, but it is always in a similar spot
in the hedge and nest building usually begins in late
February. This year, however, both the male and female
began gathering dry grass stalks, mud and moss from
around the garden in mid-March, several weeks
later than usual. I think this must be because of
the harsh late winter weather. Now, in April,
the pair have begun to collect small worms and
insect life from our patch every few minutes, a sign

that their brood has started to hatch. This simple, good thought in the midst of weeks of illness is very welcome, although I long for a little of their relentless energy and verve. The male blackbird's attempts to chase away jays remain loud and purposeful, but still futile. In the hierarchy of garden birds, the male blackbird is king only until the moment that a corvid lands on his patch.

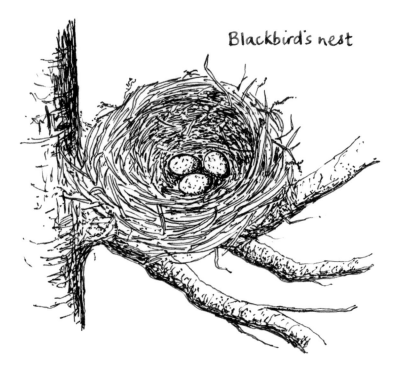

Blackbird's nest

Starlings have begun to discover our bird cafe in some numbers, and often descend in a squawky squabbly rabble to fight over mealworms and chunks of fat ball. The blackbird's ire at their presence in the garden is explosive. Each starling is slightly smaller than the blackbird, so if one flies down to the feeding station he makes short work of

their visit with a shrill ornithological diatribe and a great
deal of flapping. Starlings en masse pose more of a problem.
Sometimes he attempts to tackle them one at a time, but
this squanders energy that he needs to find worms, so on
most of their visits he opts for staring and alarm-tweeting
at them, the equivalent of bird cluster swearing, while
continuing to forage for his brood.

I grew up in suburban Liverpool where few swallows
summered. The sight of a swallow, swift or martin,
even late in the season when they have been here for
several months and have bred, has always made me feel
exhilarated. I realized early in life that these small dark
voyagers were special birds, messengers of hope, heralds of
warmer days.

Since we moved to the edge of the Fens in 2003 I have
noticed swallows arriving annually between the 12th and
14th of April, but this year these dates pass with no sign of
them. The seasons seem suspended and I feel perplexed by
their absence. I take to Twitter for a possible explanation.
Swallows have been spotted on the south coast but are
arriving weeks later than usual. There is consternation
among birders: surely, global warming should bring them
here from Africa earlier in the year. The icy weather in
March should not have affected them. What is happening?
Where are they? There is talk of bad weather in Morocco
and a delay in migration. I watch the skies. I sit in the
garden and hope that a swallow might manifest itself. There
are chattering house sparrows in the hedge, the ever-vigilant
male blackbird and a quietly careful dunnock hopping

among my viola plants, but no tail streamers, no swooping swimming flight. Long-tailed tits arrive in the garden in companionable twos and threes. They alight on the feeders and have small meals unperturbed by my presence nearby. They are a cheering sight but my eyes return to the sky, watchful for the bird I yearn to see.

As the month progresses and the temperature rises, I begin to spend more time in the garden. My recovery is slow but the soothing effects of being among plants, whether wild or cultivated, are marked. On sunny mornings I weed the flowerbeds and think about how contact with beneficial bacteria in the soil, specifically *Mycobacterium vaccae* and possibly other strains that have not yet been discovered, can shift the balance of neurotransmitters in my brain. Gardening is satisfying and gently uplifting, like mucky yoga, and along with watching the birds who visit the garden it is helping me to alleviate depressive thoughts. I remove shoots of ground elder, bindweed and the occasional thistle from a bed I have sown with flowers for cutting, to bring into the house later in the year, and I rest for a moment with a cup of tea. My eyes move skyward and there it is: the first swallow. It is swooping above the garden like a tiny blue-black dolphin in waves of air. It follows the line of the hedge where gnats and other flying insects gather, skims over the roof of the shed, dips low when it reaches the crab-apple tree and continues to mark the outline of our small patch of land, ending by landing on our old TV aerial to take a rest. It has travelled here from

South Africa, flying around two hundred miles a day on its near month-long journey of between five and six thousand miles. It is a mind-boggling feat for such a small bird. To see swallows as symbols of persistence in the face of seemingly insurmountable tasks is a cliché, but their journeys really are remarkable. Many die in storms or through predation on the way, yet most arrive, pair off, nest, lay eggs, rear young and move above the summer fields like agile feathered darts before they gather on telephone lines and leave for another year. They are here during the months of the year that I am usually well. I am so thrilled to see this bird resting on our house after its gargantuan journey. It has reached its destination and I have survived another winter. I have a small cry on the patio.

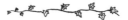

The whole family, including Annie, take a trip to Bradfield Woods. This is a very special place: an ancient patch of woodland near Bury St Edmunds that has been a working hazel coppice since the thirteenth century.

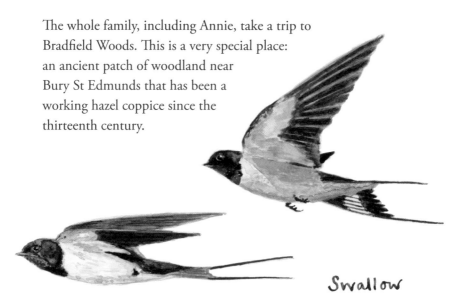

Swallow

The products of coppicing can still be bought at the entrance of the wood: pea sticks and poles for fencing and staking. Coppicing maintains open glades within the wood where wildflowers can flourish, simultaneously allowing dense thickets of honeysuckle, bramble and rose to build up, which provide the perfect habitat and cover in which nightingales can breed. This is now a rare scene in Britain – a glimpse of another age.

There has been rain and the paths are thickly sticky with mud. Puddles lie here and there, and it is bitterly cold, but beneath the coppiced hazels and along the edges of the paths the ground is peppered with botanical signs of spring. We have barely entered the wood before we see the wood anemones. These are diminutive star-like wild cousins of the jewel-coloured anemones that appear in florists in March, and the pink and white Japanese anemones that bloom in gardens in August. One of their colloquial names is smellfox, due to the musky odour of their leaves. Drifts of them grow here at Bradfield, studding the glades with floral constellations. They are living up to that other moniker of theirs, windflower, as they tremble and dance in the biting April wind. Their leaves are serrated, geranium-like and delicate, and the corolla of stamens within the single row of white petals is so perfect that I could easily lose hours gazing at these plants.

We turn a corner in the wood and a long straight ride opens up ahead of us. The going is slow: the mud is thick here – there are footprints of muntjac deer and of birds, and Annie sniffs each one, fascinated. A few metres along this woodland way I see a subtle flash of yellow and stop to examine it. An oxlip is opening its flowers. They grow at just a few sites in East Anglia. It has the petal

Wood anemones at Bradfield Woods >

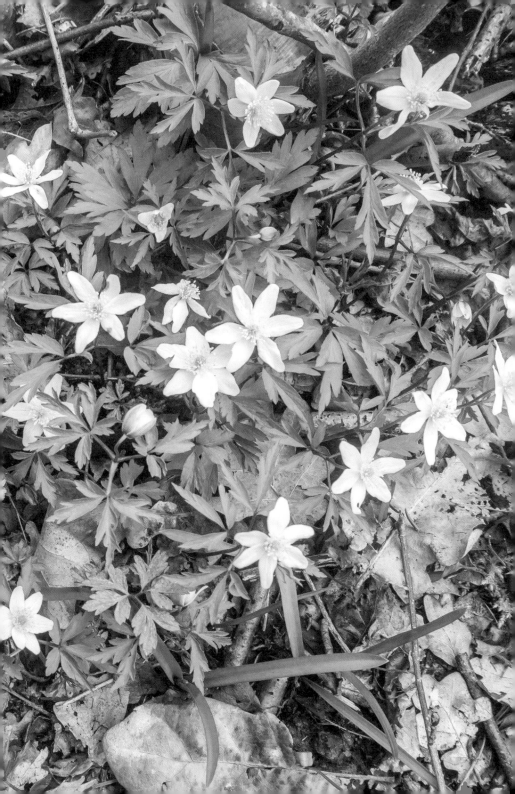

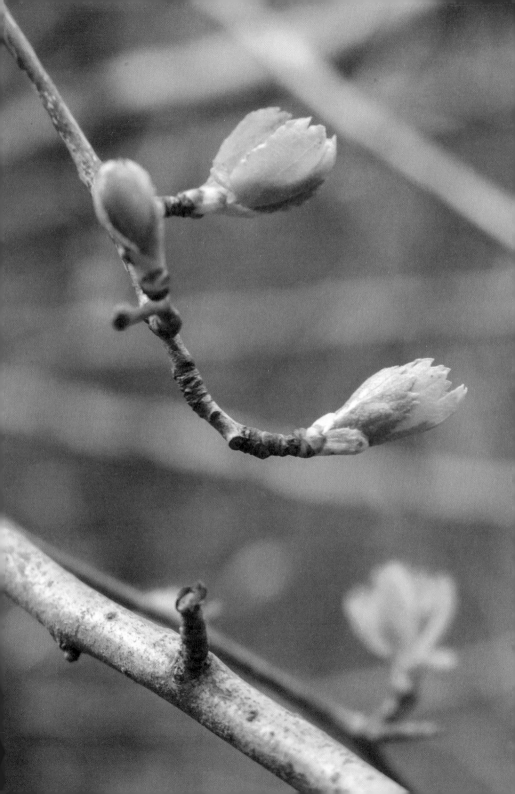

colour and flower shape of a primrose but the growing habit of a cowslip. Its stems are upright, emerging from a rosette of beautifully wrinkled leaves, and several flowers are produced at the top of each one. This flower was immortalized by Oberon's monologue in *A Midsummer Night's Dream*. The bank he speaks of where the wild thyme grows is a tangle of oxlips, eglantine (wild rose) and woodbine (honeysuckle). The botanist in me worries a little that wild thyme prefers a warm sandy soil and that oxlip grows in the cool clay-rich leaf litter of woodland, but I'd be guilty of joyless plantsplaining. There is wild honeysuckle here, winding around the coppiced hazel poles, and thickets of briar hide the nests of nightingales. Oberon speaks of a fairy bank, a glorious magical muddle of plants on which Titania likes to take her flower-scented naps. His words could have been inspired by the glades of Bradfield Woods.

The wild garlic leaves have begun to expand and the flower buds are visible. I know that one of my favourite flowers, water avens, grows along the banks of the ditches here at Bradfield. I cannot yet make them out, but I do spot the young leaves of meadowsweet, deeply concertinaed along their main veins, like botanical origami. Spring has been slowed but it is here, despite the cold and rain. I show my daughters each plant, tell them how rare the oxlips are, and they are rapt. Just as we are leaving, my youngest daughter notices a small patch of acid green above us. This year's hazel leaves are emerging. These patches of sharp bright colour against the browns and greys of the remains of winter are tiny, yet they are a wonderful sight. We leave this enchanting wood and I know that the spring signs we have seen have helped with my recovery.

‹ New hazel leaves at Bradfield Woods

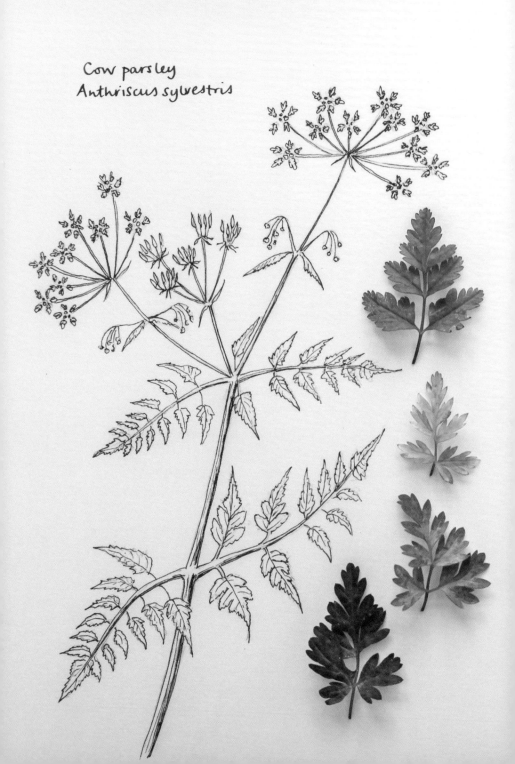

Cow parsley
Anthriscus sylvestris

May

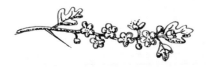

Nightingales return.
Cow parsley blooms.

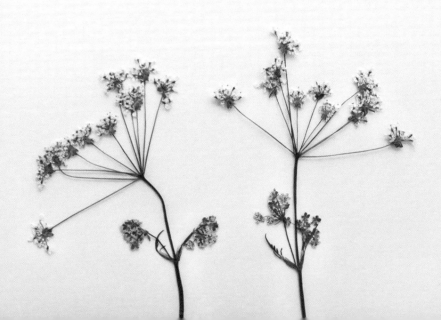

It is two months since I became unwell, and although I have lifted out of the worst of this bout of depression the shadow of low mood still lurks in my consciousness. However, as May begins, my instinct to seek out natural wonders that had been suppressed begins to reawaken. It is muffled at first but I am relieved that it has returned.

While I was ill I stayed indoors and missed a significant part of the spring, but the slowing of the seasons means that cow parsley flowers have only just begun to emerge and bluebells are at their peak now, in early May. I am pleased that I haven't missed them. The vestiges of depression are still clawing at my motivation and energy, but my compulsion to see that ethereal mist of blue on a woodland floor is too powerful for the melancholy to subdue it, so, once again, I drive to Bradfield Woods.

As I enter the wood there is that particular gentle warmth that comes when the skies clear and the spring gathers pace. The balmy weather combines with the leaf-dappled shade,

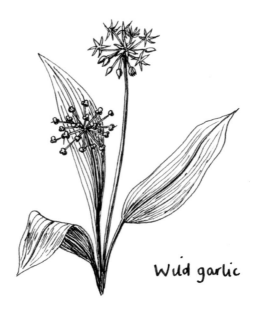

Wild garlic

the heady jumble of greens and the delicious scents of leaf
litter, spring growth and bluebells to create a cocktail of
sensory delight as I walk. This place, now, is sublime and
all of it – sunlight, scents, colours and more than that,
something of nature itself humming in the newly emerged
bees, the delicate fronds of pignut and the orchestra of
birdsong above me – sends my spirits swooping upwards.
I feel as though I want to swim in the wood's bright new
foliage, dive down into the gently mouldering layers of
last year's leaves where a wood-wide-web of fungal mycelia
connects the tree roots, and up into the glades where the
green-gold spring sunlight pours down on the wild garlic. I
stand and look and allow myself to drink in the joy of this
wood. I know there are dormice here, nightingales, orchids.
It is a potent place. A place that can heal.

I make my way to the first clearing, just metres from
the visitors' centre. Here, coppiced hazels stand, bristling
thickly with poles of growth just a few years old. A small
sign reads 'Keep off the bank, solitary bees nesting': such
a glorious sentence and evidence of the care that Suffolk
Wildlife Trust are taking of this precious habitat. I notice
small movements above the low sandy slope in front of
me. These are female tawny mining bees, a bright coppery
species, busily digging holes in which to lay their eggs,
hovering in front of their entrances and going about their

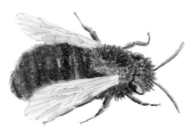

Tawny mining bee

important bee business. I saw these bees a year ago on just such a day as this. I remember watching them for an hour or more while my children built an excellent den with the hazel poles that had been harvested in the preceding winter months. I want to *know* the bees, learn how they dig these tiny burrows, and follow them on their foraging flights. I watch them for a while, spellbound.

Beyond the bank is the plant I have come to see. The flowers are at their peak: the lower bells are open, the petals of each curved backwards, and the upper bells are still in bud. The blue is deep, intense, luminous, and these flowers thrum with colour. I find a patch of ground among them covered by a tangle of wood avens, wood anemone and pignut, and sit cross-legged and gaze at them, allowing the combination of sunlight and floral abundance to enter my eyes and reach my brain. The feeling is as effective at spreading contentment as a slab of the most delicious chocolate cake or a plate of homemade chips sprinkled with salt. It is as though my mind is eating this scene and gaining sustenance from it.

The sound of solitary bees visiting the bluebells to collect nectar and pollen is soporific. I feel a pull to lie down and sleep here among the flowers. I allow time to drift. *This* is forest bathing. I am totally immersed in my surroundings: I can smell the leaf mould, the gentle scent of the bluebells; the sun is warming the back of my neck; I can hear the busy rustlings of small mammals in the undergrowth and the song of birds above me. The wood is lowering my blood pressure, lifting my

Bluebells at Bradfield Woods ›

mood and dialling down my levels of stress. There is no doubt that it is aiding my recovery. I don't know how long I stay among the bluebells, but when I leave for home I do so reluctantly.

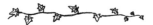

There is a junction near Fordham whose verges have been sown with native grassland wildflower species for the last three years, to create a meadow skirting the place where articulated lorries turn and cars pass by constantly on their way to Soham, Ely or Newmarket. There is no footpath through this patch of ground. In fact, I doubt many people notice it as they drive to their destination. It may register only as a very brief blur of colour, a smudge of white and yellow and purple on green. Sometimes a dented hubcap lies at the edge of it. Here and there are cigarette butts and plastic bottles among the grass, thrown from vehicles as they pass. It is an unlikely place for nature to thrive: verges nearby often become parched in summer and are sometimes sprayed with weed killer or strimmed, yet here either a landowner or the council has created a haven for insects. It is an abundant mass of species: wild marjoram, knapweed, oxeye daisy, hedge and lady's bedstraw, vetches, clover, sainfoin, hogweed and scabious. Today, the sward is bristling with cowslips. They're usually at their peak in mid- to late-April, but the effects of the snow that fell in March are still evident in the botanical calendar.

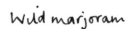

Wild marjoram

I park my car in the entrance to an abandoned
industrial estate near the railway track and walk towards
the roundabout. The cowslips are all about me: hundreds,
perhaps thousands of them creating a cloud of yellow. The
colour of cowslips is intense: a deep egg-yolk printed with
five orange spots within. Each of their five petals are heart-
shaped, giving a fluted appearance to the small open whorls
protruding from each set of sepals. It is early evening and
the sight of these flowers illuminated from behind by low
sunshine is truly beautiful. I sit here among the cowslips
as I did among the bluebells and drink in this delicately
beautiful scene in this improbable place. Vehicles roar by
just a few metres away from me but I hardly notice them.

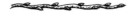

There are particular wildlife species that I try to seek out
each year: wild snake's head fritillaries in spring, gatherings
of starlings in winter, and orchids in early summer. In May
my thoughts revolve around a particular bird, an elusive
migrant, a now rare species that makes arguably one of the
most astonishing sounds of any animal. There are sequences
in its call that sound like running, bubbling water, almost
unbearably sweet repeated high notes interspersed with
trills, chromatic scales and low bass notes that audibly
mimic an engine. When I hear a nightingale's song it is as
though all my other senses are muted. My hearing takes
over and the sounds made by the bird trigger corresponding
bursts of neuronal excitement in my mind.

Nine years ago, a nightingale sang in our village wood:
the same wood I walk in with Annie most days. I could
hear it when I opened our bathroom window and was

so thrilled that I made a recording of it and posted it on my blog. Sadly, this male, who may have been aiming for Wicken Fen when he alighted among the young trees behind our cottage in 2009, neither found a mate nor returned the following year.

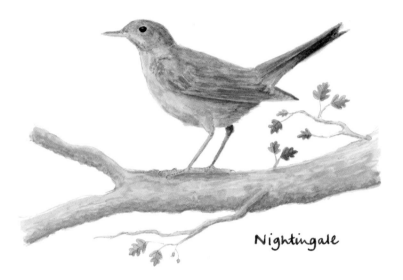

Nightingale

My urge to hear nightingales is so strong that I have driven for an hour and a half to go on nightingale walks in a place called Glapthorn Cow Pastures, a pocket of dense protected woodland in Northamptonshire. I have held unsuccessful one-woman vigils on a picnic rug at Wicken Fen, straining to hear the very few birds that return there each year. I heard tens of nightingales in Tuscany calling across a wooded valley, and it was one of the most exquisite and important nature-based experiences of my life. I am keen to find nightingales closer at hand, though, so I scour the internet for nearby breeding sites and come across Lackford Lakes near Bury St Edmunds. Apparently, several pairs breed there and it is just half an hour away along the A14.

One evening I set off at around 7 p.m. and arrive at Lackford Lakes car park as dusk is falling. The light is soft, the sky an ombre of subdued blues, and towards the horizon the blues blend seamlessly into a band of delicate primrose yellow. The silhouettes of the spring trees, newly in leaf, make intricate filigree patterns against the evening light. I park my car and open the window. Immediately my ears are met with a wall of birdsong. This is the evening chorus, a time when many species of bird will find a high perch and proclaim their territory in spring. I can see bird shapes in silhouette on the highest branches of the trees surrounding the car park. It is an ornithological choir that sings out a beautiful warning: a simultaneous proclamation by each bird that they are here and have a nest, a family, so do not dare trespass on their territory.

As the light falls further, the chorus diminishes, leaving the late singing stalwarts, blackbird and song thrush, carolling loudly from the tops of surrounding trees. Beneath the fluting call of the blackbird and the repeated stanzas of the song thrush there is another song. It is barely audible, so I lock my car and walk towards it. The blackbirds have begun to settle for the night: they are still singing but more time elapses between each of their verses until eventually they fall silent. The song thrushes are now quiet and are roosting. Some of the notes of the remaining song are muffled by the distance and by the dense undergrowth, but a low, distinct 'chug-chug-chug' sequence marks it out as a nightingale. As soon as I recognize it I stop and listen intently, allowing the sound to coalesce and take form in my ears. Exquisite repeated high

notes that seem plaintive, as though the bird is expressing
some intense emotion that is almost unbearable, sound
out through the trees. These notes unlock my thoughts
unexpectedly. The winter was long, life was tough during
those months, and my mind paid the price. I'm only just
beginning to feel alive again. The nightingale's song tumbles
from some distant invisible point among the trees and it
seems to snap these things into focus. Each time depression
catches me I fight it with all the armoury I have, just about
wriggle free, recover slowly and try to continue with life.
The cycle is inexorable and exhausting but I stay firmly in
that day; I do not think of the illness as a whole. Standing
here listening to this intricate beautiful sound, the thoughts
that I suppress suddenly erupt in my mind. I realize that
it's unlikely that I'll ever be free of my condition and
that it has burgled my ability to enjoy life fully for more
than half of my life. I realize that I detest my depression.
It sits on my mind like a great grey mollusc and I punch
my way from beneath it whenever I can, hit out at it by
being among trees, among birds and plants, I trample it by
diverting my mind into the more positive states that can
come when I draw, paint or make things with my hands.
I seek talking cures, take medicine daily, increase the dose
if the darkness becomes overwhelming. I have to rest and
sleep far more than I want to, and am unable to achieve
as much as I would like. It is a never-ending task to try to
keep this condition in check, a miserable *magnum opus*.
I'm tired and suddenly long for a short holiday from it:
just one day when I can wake and simply enjoy what I am
doing without having to diminish my expectations of what
is possible. I cry there at Lackford Lakes while listening
to a small rare bird producing a lovely song. I stand and

let the tears come. I sob and snot falls from my nose onto
the path. I allow the hatred and anger I feel to come out
messily and noisily. Then I wrench my mind back to reality,
put these thoughts back in their ghastly mental box, get
back in my car and drive home.

The next day I feel well. Allowing myself to
acknowledge how exhausting it is to live with depression
has left my mind feeling lighter. I put Annie on her lead
and walk up to the wood behind the cottage. We take
our usual route, and the familiar paths we follow through
the trees are reassuring. The wood smells delicious. Elder
and hawthorn have come into flower and the sharp-sweet
muscat scents they emit mix with the mushroom odour
of leaf litter and the intense smell of green – of lush grass
and innumerable plants in full leaf. I stop to examine
some hawthorn blossom. Each small five-petalled flower
is exquisite and there are hundreds of thousands of them
garlanding this tree, emitting an intoxicating scent. I think
of the haw berries that will begin to develop in a few weeks.
Their intense claret colour is a kind of vivid visual medicine
for me. For three out of the four seasons, hawthorn is
able to soothe my mind and help to fend off mental
darkness, and I feel intensely grateful
towards this tree. As I stand there
inhaling the blossom's heady scent,
I think of Nan Shepherd's words
about pine trees: 'When the
aromatic savour … goes searching
into the deepest recesses of my
lungs, I know it is life that is
entering. I draw life in through
the delicate hairs of my nostrils.'

Elderflower

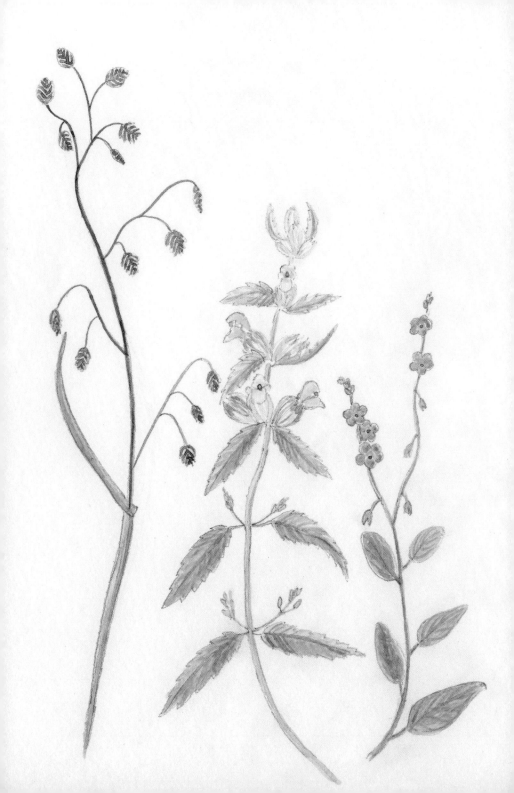

June

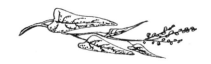

Meadow browns emerge.
Bee orchids bloom.

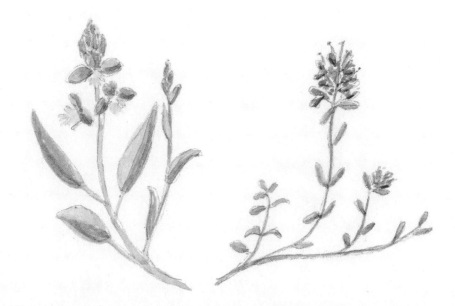

The conveyor belt of flowering plants that began with snowdrops in February has gone into overdrive. Early in the year the progression is always slow, with the snowdrops and aconites followed in late February by cherry plum blossom, blackthorn, dog's mercury, wild daffodils and wood anemone. In March and April, the frequency steps up a little and becomes pleasingly steady. I am able to absorb each species fully as it appears: examine it, savour it, photograph, draw and press it (if it is common enough), and when the flowers cease I mourn a little but can then focus on another as it takes its turn. In May and June, the rate of growth of the plants in both hedgerow and garden becomes dizzyingly fast. Provided there is sufficient rain between the warm spells, the verdure in hedgerows shifts from tentative growth to an exuberant lushness.

It is mid-May and the cow parsley leaves reach maturity and the flower spikes begin to fizz upwards like subtle botanical fireworks. This is the point in the year when I begin to lose track of the emergence of flowers: ground ivy, pignut, white deadnettle, yellow archangel, hawthorn, hawkbits, wood avens, borage, field poppy, hedge bedstraw, lady's bedstraw, hogweed and countless others, all flowering at once and overlapping, tumbling into bloom, filling the verges with so many flowers I barely know how to take them all in. May

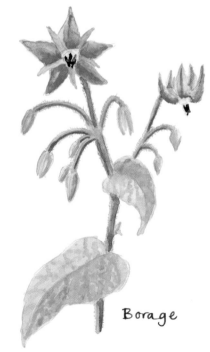

Borage

is so starkly different in terms of plant growth to January that it is like another botanical country and yet they are only ninety days apart. June is the time when I begin to wish the year would slow down. I want to stretch the growing season out, so that I might more easily absorb the green abundance of the weeks ahead of midsummer, before the grasses start to become bleached and brown and the year steers towards autumn. I want to press pause.

As I watch the hawthorn blossom fade (a small sadness), observe the cow parsley that has gone to seed (until next year, favourite flower), see the field poppies bleed along the selvedges of farmland (please stay awhile) and the first elderflowers begin to turn brown (oh bloody hell, this year is going too fast), an idea strikes me. I can't press pause, but perhaps I can rewind … by travelling north. Perhaps I can chase spring up the country. This thought simmers in my mind for a week or two and I begin to wonder where I could go.

On Twitter I see images of the diminutive hardy flora growing in the crevices (grykes) of the limestone pavement of Hutton Roof: perhaps I should go to Lancashire. That infamous app, so renowned for embittered e-battles and bile, has gentler corners that show me tantalizing pictures of delicate British orchids: fly, green-winged, common spotted, bee, southern marsh and delicate twayblades. My desire to see orchids and, perhaps, cow parsley that is still in bloom, becomes overwhelming and I settle on Derbyshire as a place to seek them out. There are several meadows in that county that have never been treated with fertilizers. The Derbyshire Wildlife Trust website speaks of 'orchids' and 'abundance', and urges readers to visit the meadows in June when the flora is at its peak. I find a minuscule cottage for rent on Airbnb and set out one evening in the second week of the month.

The next morning, before I leave the little stone house I have rented near Bakewell, I read about Rose End Meadows in Cromford, and find a few slightly grainy pictures online of lush green sward pinpricked with pale pink orchids. I follow the directions from my sat nav and end up in a housing estate. Can this be right? Am I on a wild goose chase? I doubt my research and look dazedly at my phone. Sure enough the postcode is among a hundred or more friendly-looking houses clinging to the hill. I strike out, determined to find the meadows, and ask someone leaning over their garden wall if they are nearby. 'You're in the right place,' she says. 'Just follow those steps upwards and keep left. You'll find it.' It still seems implausible that a nature reserve should be so close to a densely populated area and that I might see orchids here, but I scale the steps and at the top is a grass path bristling on one side with hawkbits, cow parsley that has gone to seed and towering thistles. The other side of the path is lined with the walls of back gardens. The way winds around a corner, up a short, steep incline with thick tree roots protruding from the ground, and there on my right is a gate and a sign telling me I have reached Rose End Meadows. The distance between this secluded entrance and the back gardens I left behind is only a few metres. No gentle transition, this: my surroundings have shifted abruptly from glimpses of garden ponds, toddler tricycles and whiffs of frying bacon to a place that is headily bucolic. The gate is surrounded by elder coming into flower, hawthorn bearing embryonic berries bows from the other side of the path to meet it, and at my feet is a verdant muddle of red campion, green alkanet and starbursts of hogweed flowers.

This feeling of being on a threshold, of following a path into an unknown place, of potentially finding something that I have been seeking, makes me feel slightly light-headed. I am an embarrassingly unworldly person. I barely travelled at all when I was young due to illness and lack of confidence, and circumstances, have prevented my small family from venturing abroad since I became a mother twelve years ago, but small local or UK-based adventures, seeking out new habitats, rare plants or modest wildlife spectacles, are as wondrous to me as any sighting of a crocodile, condor or canyon. I'm thrilled to be in this place.

I open the gate. The path climbs steeply and is lined on each side by solid green verges so that for several seconds I am unable to see further than a metre or two in any direction. Then the way levels out and to my right the land pitches steeply away into a small clearing, edged with mature sycamores and hawthorn and peppered thickly with hogweed flowers emerging from dense grasses. To my left the meadow forms a near horizon. I am in rolling country and this plot of grassland is clinging to the slopes like the botanical version of an Italian hill town.

I look towards my feet and immediately see a jumble of plants, several of which I have only ever seen in reference books. There are large swathes of ground covered in very low-growing species, like a meadowland version of the

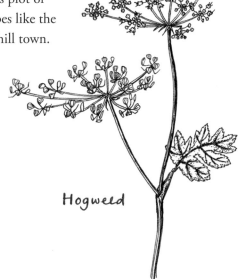

Hogweed

lichen heath I saw at Dungeness. Breckland thyme no more than 3 cm tall is in flower, and scattered among sprawling cushions of it are constellations of minuscule floral stars resembling tiny white harebells. A dim memory is sparked in my mind and a quick Google search confirms that this is fairy flax. It strikes me as I search the internet in this wild place that my phone is the equivalent of carrying several botanical reference books with me. I wonder what Victorian naturalists such as Anna Atkins, exponent of cyanotypes and passionate seaweed fanatic, would make of the contraption I rely on to identify plant species.

I have grown common flax in my garden. It's an elegant ethereal plant with intensely blue five-petalled flowers, similar to those my daughters drew when they were small, each of which lasts just twenty-four hours. The flowers of this miniature wild flax are breathtakingly delicate and the sight of this plant, a new species for me and one whose uses I have read about (purging and poultices) gives me a burst of elation that could perhaps be called a nature-spotting or naturalist's high. Then

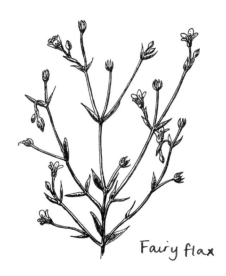

Fairy flax

a small patch of blue catches my eye and a plant I have longed to see is just there in front of my shoes. Once my mind has attuned to this new thrill I spy strands of it among the thyme and fairy flax for several metres in all directions. This is milkwort. Around 7 cm tall, it is the blue of delphiniums and clear Caribbean skies, and within the outer petals is a delicate white fringe like the tail of a tiny albino peacock. It prefers chalky ground, was traditionally used to treat respiratory complaints, and Keble Martin painted it growing among wild rocket, sea kale and rock rose on Plate 11 of *The Concise British Flora in Colour*. The botany of this place is Lilliputian, but the exhilaration it triggers in me is intense. My brain floods with dopamine, and I know there are more benign highs to be had, so I continue to explore.

I clamber towards the hogweed in the clearing to my right and the botany changes from low-lying, dry, delicate heath to a tangle of lush grasses. The childhood reflex to sit in long grass and among flowers has never left me, so I do just that. Many of the grasses' seed heads reach my shoulders and I feel like a wild mammal using vegetation to hide myself. I begin to examine the plant life around me. I soon spot yellow rattle, a semi-parasitic plant that gains some of its nutrients from the roots of grasses growing nearby. This plant can dramatically increase the botanical diversity of a meadow habitat by suppressing the growth of invasive grass species and allowing a wider range of wildflowers and other plants to colonize. I see grass seed heads that resemble very small squat oats and realize, with a further burst of botanical delight, that this is quaking grass – another species I have longed to see since I was very young. A zephyr-like breeze moves through the meadow and the quaking grass shivers and trembles, the seed heads seeming to dance in the air on their hair-fine stalks like tiny puppet bees.

Here and there, small hawthorns are growing among the meadow plants. Their presence must alter the soil because around their roots the flora is different and has a hint of woodland rather than open hay meadow about it: red campion, alkanet, forget-me-nots with one or two flowers remaining, and the small spiky seed heads of wood avens. I approach one of the hawthorns to take a closer look at the place where one habitat meets another and there in front of me is an orchid. It is a delicate pale pink, rather small, just 10 cm high, and utterly exquisite. The flower spikes of most British orchids are inflorescences: several small flowers grouped on a single stalk. Each individual flower of this orchid resembles that of a lobelia and has five petals intricately patterned with deep cerise spots and strokes. The flowers are clustered at the top of the stalk to form a shape like a tiny floral teepee. At its apex, each flower is tightly in bud, and at its base they are in full bloom. I wonder if there are more specimens nearby and scan the few metres surrounding me.

These are common spotted-orchids, *Dactylorhiza fuchsii*, one of the most prevalent species in the UK. Three or four more orchids are growing among the quaking grass and yellow rattle. Each species of wild orchid has a symbiotic relationship with a specific fungal species, without which they would be unable to germinate. The pH, friability and microbiome of the soil and the microclimate of the surrounding

Common spotted-orchid at Rose End Meadows, Derbyshire ›

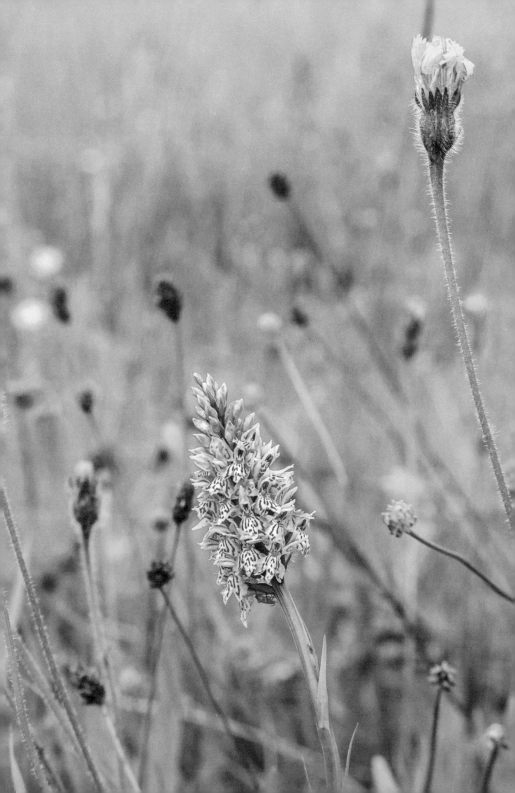

habitat have to be just right in order for both organisms to thrive. This orchid species is small and subtle and could easily be overlooked, yet its presence is a sign that this land at Rose End Meadows is the antithesis of the sterile fields of grain that cover so much of our country. This place is not just rich in plant life; beneath the soil, microorganisms and fungi are interacting with each other and with the plants, and those relationships form a complex interwoven web that underpins this meadow and permits it to exist. The thought that so much of our country was once this rich in biodiversity is chastening. The wonder I feel at this small patch of uncontaminated soil and its lush riot of flowers and grasses is tinged with a longing for a wilder Britain, one that existed centuries ago, before we permitted industrial intensive farming to consume our meadows, before this land of ours became a factory.

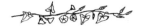

I have been searching for the leaves of bee orchids in the village wood since the autumn. They are smallish, slender, and at first glance – among an assortment of wild carrot, black medick, field maple saplings, clover and grasses – can easily be mistaken for the leaves of plantain. I know they grow in the wood because I've seen them almost every year since we arrived here in 2003, but the places in which they appear are slightly different each time. This could be because each individual plant does not flower every year and new specimens germinate, giving the impression of a small population that moves about among the trees. One or two bee orchids used to grow just inside the wood along a slender muntjac path to the left-hand side of the main route. However, this area of wood has become overgrown in recent years. Orchids prefer direct or dappled sunlight and cannot thrive in areas with low light levels and I have not been able to find any orchids here in the last two years. There is another place on the edge of the wood, near where I found the ladybirds hibernating among knapweed seed heads, where one or two bee orchids sometimes emerge in the grasses along the edge of the path, but I cannot always find them and I fear that they may be beheaded when the paths are mown.

My youngest daughter and I decide to go on an orchid hunt. First, we walk to the edge of the meadow near the patch of lichen-encrusted hawthorn where I discovered several bee orchid flower spikes last year. We find wild carrot in bud, drifts of clover and a tangle of vetches, but no orchids. We search along the path that skirts the wood, but again find none. My daughter has brought a small net with her that she uses to catch shrimps and crabs when we go rockpooling. In the summer months she uses it to try to catch butterflies, and for a little while we forget about the orchids as we hunt for our flying quarry: meadow browns, common blues, small heaths, speckled woods and large whites. She catches them gently in the mesh of the net so

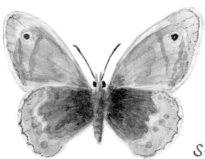

Small heath

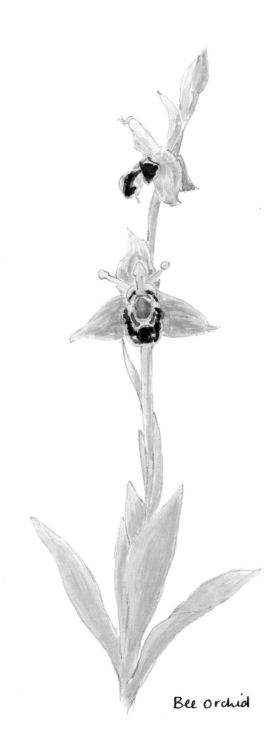

Bee Orchid

that she can examine them closely, and once she has taken in their colouring and learned the pattern on their wings in order to be able to recognize them again, she lets them go. In truth, she only manages to capture one or two, as she's worried about damaging their wings, but it is a pastime we both love and we lose track of time.

It is midsummer, the sun is hot on our backs and I begin to crave a cold drink, so we make our way towards home. Suddenly, next to the path where a dense patch of wild carrot grows and where I saw the flock of long-tailed tits in December, I spy a bee orchid in flower. I have never seen one in this spot before and I explain to my daughter how the astonishing flower shape originally evolved to attract real bees (specifically the solitary bee *Eucera*) to try to mate with the flowers and carry pollen from plant to plant. Apart from some populations in the Mediterranean, bee orchids now propagate by self-pollination, but she is enchanted and squats down to examine the flower for some time.

'The wings of the orchid bee are pink!' she exclaims. 'I would love to see a bee with pink wings.'

'So would I,' I reply, and we walk home, stopping once or twice on the way to try to catch a small tortoiseshell butterfly that is basking on the path.

Field
poppy

Wild
fennel

Toadflax

Corn
chamomile

July

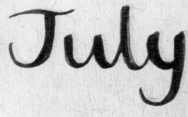

Wild carrot blooms.
Burnet moths emerge.

Common
flax

Common
Knapweed

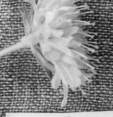

Field
Scabious

As a result of being ill in March and April, my social confidence seems to have dwindled. My urge to hide away from even close friends is far stronger than it was a year ago and I realize that I have become semi-reclusive. This is a common effect of depression and can manifest itself in a slowly creeping, insidious way. If the black dog is lurking in my brain, the self-diminishing thoughts that accompany it make venturing out of the house and engaging in conversation seem daunting. Depression convinces me that I have nothing interesting to say, that there is very little point in going out and that it is easier to *not* make plans with friends. This is another form of anhedonia. Depression steals a person's ability to enjoy all aspects of life, and when it affects social interaction the result is isolation. This erodes social confidence further: it is a vicious circle that can be difficult to break, strengthening the hold that the illness has on the mind. I make the excuse to myself that I have work to do, illustrations to complete, and that I don't have time to see friends, but if I am honest I know that depriving myself of good company and laughter is a lingering effect of what happened in the spring.

July begins with searing heat. It becomes almost uncomfortable to be outdoors and I take fewer walks. There is more bright sunshine during these first weeks of July than I can remember in several years but, while for some people just the sight of a sunny day through a window can make a difference, its mood-lifting effects can really only be felt if it hits the retina or skin directly. I hide indoors away from the heatwave as though it were January. The combined effects of self-isolation and the urge to stay in the cottage's coolish interior have resulted in a feeling of disconnection from the world. I realize that the longer I permit these hermit-like urges to dominate, the trickier it will be to begin socializing again.

It is a tweet that sparks me into action. Glow-worms have been spotted at Wicken Fen just a few miles from our village. I text my friend and fellow biologist Rachael to see if she fancies a night-time search for glimmers in the hedgerows. Glow-worms are a species of beetle, and during the mating season the females illuminate their abdomens with green light produced by luciferase, a bioluminescent enzyme. Males see the females' tiny light displays and fly out to find them. It's a small saucy beetly light show. I have seen fireflies in Tuscany but I have never seen a British glow-worm. Rachael and I each bring a daughter and set out across the Fen.

Dusk has fallen as we cross the small wooden bridge to the wetland reserve at Wicken. This has the feel of an adventure about it already, and I begin to feel gleeful and relieved. For weeks I have starved myself of both company and contact with nature, and I can feel the negative effects of that deprivation beginning to lift. Almost immediately we become aware of dragonflies as long as sausages hawking along the wide mown path and flitting above our heads. The light level is low, but these are likely to be southern hawkers, one of Britain's largest species. Flying among them are moths, and I watch a dragonfly pursue one. The moth becomes aware of this agile winged assassin and drops down into the reeds to avoid it. I am already charmed by this place and we are only a few metres from the visitor centre. Our eyes skim the ground as we search for pinpricks of green light.

We reach a crossways of grassy paths among the reeds and take a left-hand turn. As we do so, a whirring starts up in a far stand of trees: a distant yet distinct sound that reminds me of a sewing machine or high-pitched drill. I realize with excitement that it might be a nightjar, whose churring mating call can be heard at this time of year in the nearby Brecklands. Nightjars are hauntingly fascinating birds: they nest on the ground and their feathers are so intricately barred and mottled that the resemblance to bark and lichen is astonishing; when they roost on a branch during the day they can become almost invisible. They have a wide pink gape, giving their faces a toad-like quality, and they perform mesmerizing crepuscular mating dances like giant moths, flitting above heath and woodland clearings in June and July while they call to one another with their mechanical-sounding vibrato. There are certain creatures, such as hares and woodlice, which have a particular appearance or behaviour that has captured the human imagination, and as a result are given nicknames steeped in affection. Nightjars fall into this category. Thirty-four colloquial names for nightjar have been gathered by the RSPB, including 'moth hawk', 'night swallow', 'razor grinder' and 'flying toad'. The word nightjar is probably derived from 'night chur', a local name that describes this bird's remarkable call. I check online and there have been no recent sightings of nightjars at Wicken, but I have heard them in Thetford Forest and this sound is identical, so I'm puzzled.

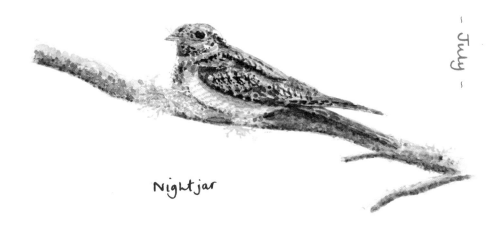

Nightjar

We had not reckoned on the mosquitoes. Rachael
has doused herself with insect repellent in an impressive
piece of forethought, but I am wearing a vest top, jeans
and sandals. A reedy high-pitched incessant whine keeps
approaching my head, and I feel an ominous tickling on
my shoulders, back and feet. I think we have become a
walking feast. There is very little light remaining and it's
impossible to see the mosquitoes, but it's easy to imagine
swarms of them. Although my skin begins to crawl, I
maintain my poise, determined to spot a glow-worm. We
decide to put a little distance between ourselves and the
main wetland area, and try searching along one of the
tracks that skirt the Fen.

Ahead of and above us in the sky is a bright point of
light as we walk along the track, and a star-gazing app
identifies it as Jupiter. As we gaze at it for a moment, two
birds fly over. There is something about the shape of their
silhouettes that makes me examine them more closely.
Both their necks and legs are almost unfeasibly long.
Geese perhaps? Or swans? No, their legs are longer than

their bodies. I check online and there have been sightings of storks at Wicken in the last week. Storks! I have always thought of them as exotic chimney-top nesters, long-legged birds of very far away. The British Trust for Ornithology estimates that there are just ten breeding pairs in Britain. I reel. This unexpected sighting of a truly rare species flying at twilight is very welcome after my recent reclusiveness. I forget the weeks I have spent cooped up and the lonely isolation I have inflicted on myself. I am in a beautiful place with a dear pal and wildlife is all around me.

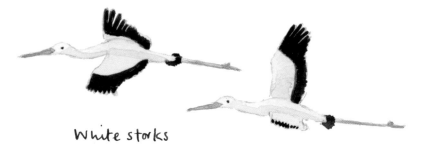

White storks

Rachael, our daughters and I make our way back to the car. We have seen no glow-worms and the mosquitoes have enjoyed a meal at our expense, but as we enter the car park I see a little owl fly towards an oak tree in the hedge: another joyful sight. It begins to call, a half-hearted sort of husky whistle, and just as it does so a man walks into the car park with a telescope. I ask what he has spotted that evening and whether he has seen any glow-worms. He hasn't but he has been watching an entire family of little owls feeding near a stack of fence posts on a track on the far side of the reserve. We listen to the owl calling from the oak, and I ask about the whirring sound we heard on the Fen. Apparently, there

have been several reports of a
nightjar at Wicken in recent
weeks.

Little
owl

We have only been here
for around half an hour, the
mosquitoes having forced us
to return to the car, so storks,
dragonflies, little owl, nightjar
is an impressive list of encounters.
My mood has changed. This brief
night adventure has made me realize quite
how far downward I had slipped, despite
it being high summer. I curse myself
for my lack of vigilance. I had stopped
actively fending off the grey slug of low
mood and it had slithered back under the
fence while my back was turned. I vow to
resume my daily walks. I need large doses
of both immersion in nature and time spent with friends,
and I need them sharpish.

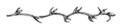

The next day the weather is so hot that spending time
outside becomes unbearable: paving stones and gravel are
far too hot to stand on in bare feet. Rachael and I have
lunch together and she tells me about the butterflies that
have been visiting her buddleias. Moving from her shady
kitchen into the garden is like plunging myself into a
furnace, but she has five buddleias in full bloom and I'm
determined to see the butterflies for myself. Immediately, I
can see three peacocks and four or five whites nectaring on

the long purple and white clusters of flowers. A red admiral flies in and I stand watching this busy insect cafe for a while, before becoming so uncomfortable in the heat that I move towards the kitchen door. As I do so, I see another large butterfly, wings closed, feeding on a flower near the top of one of the bushes. Something about the colouring and pattern of the underside of its wings ignites a memory. I realize that it might be a species I haven't spotted for two years, one I have been longing to see, and I speak to the butterfly, urging it to open its wings. Rachael asks who I am talking to and, with embarrassment, I admit that I'm conversing with an insect. The wings open and I see their upper side: at first glance it looks like a red admiral, but no, there is something different: it's as though the colour saturation has been turned down. Instead of red-black-white, it is orange-russet-white. I almost do a dance: it's a painted lady.

This insect has travelled from Morocco via Spain to settle on Rachael's buddleia here in the east of England. It is a journey of 4,500 miles undertaken to escape the butterfly's nemesis, a tiny parasitic wasp that seeks out its caterpillars and injects them with eggs. I learned about this astonishing migration from a BBC documentary about the painted lady, and have been fascinated by this species ever since. It lifts off the buddleia and flies away over the cottage roofs. I long to follow it, to witness the next stage in its life. It is a fresh specimen, with clear vivid wing patterns, and it looks as though it may be ready to mate. Painted ladies breed here in Britain in late summer and their progeny will set off back to Morocco in the autumn.

The consistent dry weather seems to have increased the numbers of both butterflies and bees across the

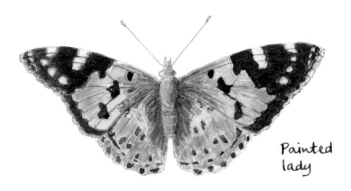

Painted lady

UK. I have never seen such numbers in our garden, on unmown roadside verges and in the wood. The use of neonicotinoids (a group of pesticides that adversely affects bee reproduction) has decreased in the last five years and I wonder if this has contributed to the apparent increase in the insect population. My observations are of a very small sample but there is more anecdotal evidence from many people, including naturalists, on Twitter. A rather gruesome piece of evidence comes in the form of increased numbers of small corpses seen on car windscreens in recent weeks, especially after travelling on motorways. Might pollinator numbers be recovering? If so, could it be due to this single season of especially dry weather? A citizen science project called The Big Butterfly Count takes place in July. I'm longing to know the results, but will have to wait several months while the statistics are being collated and dedicated volunteers do important butterfly maths.

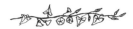

Only 3 per cent of Britain's wildflower meadows are still in place. Most have been ploughed and turned into intensively

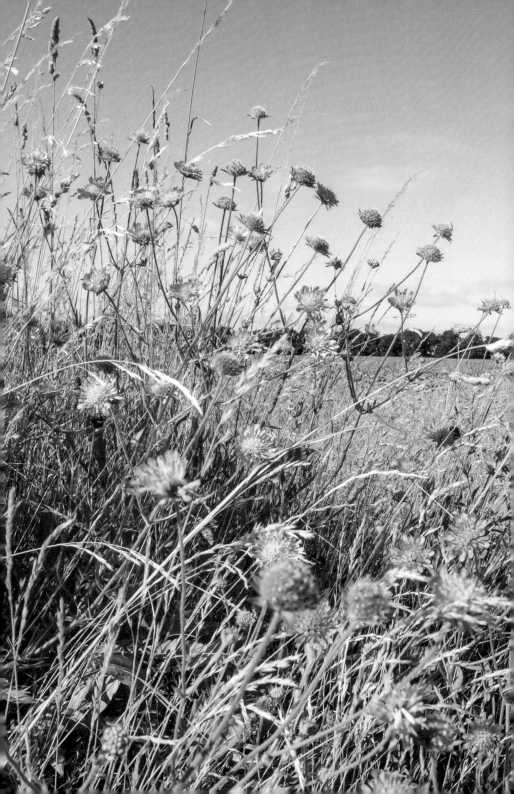

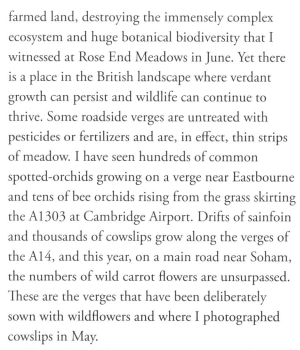

farmed land, destroying the immensely complex ecosystem and huge botanical biodiversity that I witnessed at Rose End Meadows in June. Yet there is a place in the British landscape where verdant growth can persist and wildlife can continue to thrive. Some roadside verges are untreated with pesticides or fertilizers and are, in effect, thin strips of meadow. I have seen hundreds of common spotted-orchids growing on a verge near Eastbourne and tens of bee orchids rising from the grass skirting the A1303 at Cambridge Airport. Drifts of sainfoin and thousands of cowslips grow along the verges of the A14, and this year, on a main road near Soham, the numbers of wild carrot flowers are unsurpassed. These are the verges that have been deliberately sown with wildflowers and where I photographed cowslips in May.

Today, I park the car in a gateway near the Soham bypass and walk along the thin strip of grassland that skirts the road so that I can get a better look at the profusion of flowers. Wild carrot, also called Queen Anne's lace, is a beautiful umbellifer that is used as a food source for many species of pollinator; each flattish intricate fractal-like inflorescence looks ovoid when viewed from the side and, unlike sunflowers, which orient to the sun, each wild carrot flower grows at a slightly different angle, making a drift of them seem like a highly magnified section of the night sky full of tiny floral galaxies.

On another verge, near a village called Swaffham Bulbeck, I spy a delicate mauve haze as I drive by.

< Field scabious growing by the road near Dullingham, Cambridgeshire

Field scabious flowers are growing just 30 cm or so from where the cars are passing at sixty miles an hour, making it tricky to reach them with my camera, but when I do, this mass of wildflowers is a breathtaking sight. Bees and hoverflies visiting the scabious to feed create a hum that is audible in the gaps between vehicles. As I stand in this narrow meadow, I see poppies, yarrow, hawkbits, cow parsley seed heads, Good King Henry and knapweed: a rich jumble of wildflowers among the grasses.

I wonder at this habitat, tucked in between a busy thoroughfare and vast swathes of intensely farmed land. There must be a network of many thousands of miles of these thin strips of meadow criss-crossing the country, supporting insects, passerines, raptors, owls, mammals and even reptiles through their diversity of plants. Sadly, councils or farmers often mow verges without a thought for the wildlife they support. The thirty or more bee orchids I saw springing up among oxeye daisies just metres from the perimeter fence of Cambridge Airport last year were scalped by industrial mowers before they could set seed. I wish I had informed the council that I found them. Frankly, I would have staged a sit-in to save them. I would have painted banners.

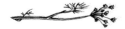

Photographs of butterflies keep appearing in my Twitter feed throughout July. A collection of shots of species I have only ever seen in reference books taken at a place called Fermyn Woods, just over an hour's drive away, are too tantalizing to ignore.

The walk between my car and the Fermyn Woods visitor

centre doesn't seem to hold much promise for wildlife
sightings. There is a large play area of sandpits, swings and
climbing frames, and an entire nursery of toddlers is sitting
on the grass eating their sandwiches and chattering happily.
This is a lovely sight, but surely a place that provides such
an excellent space for children to play in cannot also be a
habitat for unusual wildlife. I am wrong about this. Just
a few metres further is a place called 'the plateau', a raised
area of grassy heathland reached by a few metres' climb
up steep sandy paths. I step onto the heath and almost
immediately an insect catches my eye, flying low over the
grasses. It is a six-spot burnet moth and it comes into land
on the flower of a tall spear thistle where another six-spot
is waiting for it. They begin to mate and, as they do so, a
butterfly with black-and-white chequered wings rises from
deep among the grasses, flies over the grassy path I am
standing on and out across the plateau. It is a
marbled white, a striking species that I have
only seen once before, in the clearing of the
village wood. Within seconds of entering this
habitat I have encountered two charismatic
and beautiful insects, neither of which I have
seen so far this year.

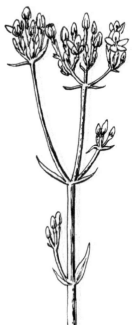

I begin to look about me and realize that
this is a place with a very different botany to
that of Rose End Meadows, but it is just as
rich. Among the grasses are yellow spikes of
agrimony, delicate stars of corn chamomile
and the beautiful pink clusters of common
centaury, a flower I have only seen on Plate
58 of Keble Martin before today. Smudges
of purple mark out knapweed in bloom

Common Centaury

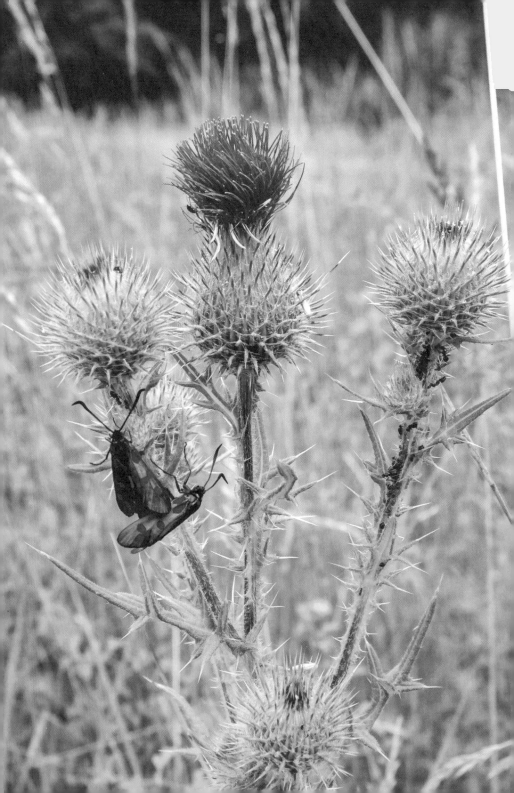

and I catch sight of cinnabar moth caterpillars on stems of ragwort, wearing their jaunty yellow-and-black stripes as though these are lepidopteran football colours. As I wander along the path, now becoming parched in the heatwave, there is a constant shimmer of wings above the vegetation: ringlets, gatekeepers, meadow browns, small heaths, Essex, small and skippers, marbled whites, and more six-spot burnets than I have ever seen before, their empty chrysalises left on grass stalks like punctuation marks. So many of the species I longed to see as a child, as I pored over my *Guide to Butterflies and Moths*, are right here in front of me that it seems like a hallucination. My mind is buoyed upwards by this place. All other thoughts dwindle to whispers as my eyes drink in each new species and the heady combination of them all jumbled into a few hundred square metres; it strikes me that this could be called heath bathing, and it is just as effective at sending my dark thoughts packing as its woodland equivalent. If only I were able to capture *this* feeling, bottle this utter joy in the presence of plants and wildlife around me when I am struck down by depression and unable to leave the house. Watching birds through our living room window in April helped to lift my depression, but that was like taking a single ibuprofen tablet for the pain of a broken leg. Fermyn Woods is like an opiate.

‹ Six-spot burnet moths mating on a spear thistle at Fermyn Woods Country Park, Northamptonshire

Cinnabar moth caterpillar

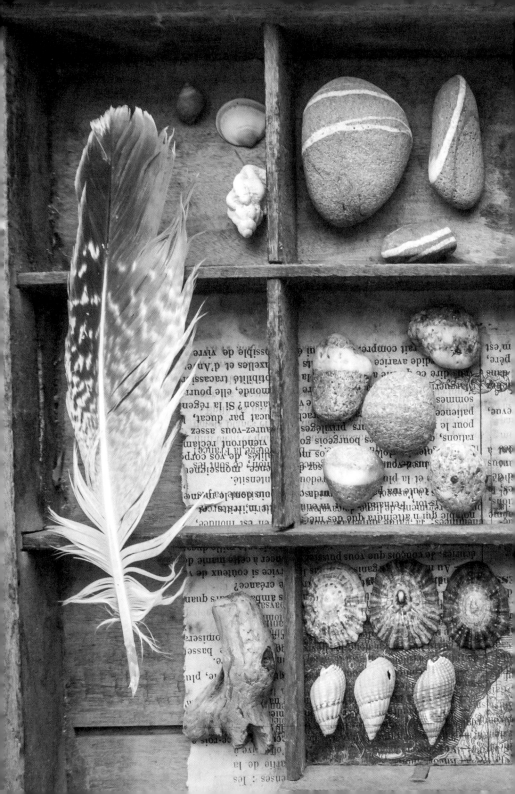

August

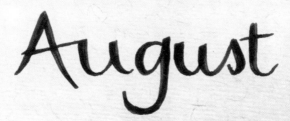

Cow parsley germinates.
Sloes ripen.

Found on
Marloes beach
(pebbles were
returned)

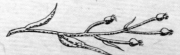

For eight consecutive years of my childhood, from the age of four, our family holidays were spent on the coast of Pembrokeshire in West Wales. The journey there from Liverpool took six hours or more, and it seemed to me to be one of the furthest-flung places on earth. Those fortnights on the Welsh coast were one of the times of the year when the family was relaxed and happy, which made them immensely precious. To my eyes, Pembrokeshire was a transformative wonderland where everything was good. We were allowed to stay up late and go on trips to the beach *after dinner*. I have memories of shops being open until dusk. People could buy things ... in the evening! This seemed terribly exotic to me – the sort of thing that happened in Spain or America. The drive back to our bed and breakfast after such night adventures was one of the best parts of these holidays. From the car window, we would see wildlife: bats, rabbits, flurries of moths, owls and, once, a badger, all going about their business. I'm not sure whether any other members of the family noticed these creatures, but I always sat up as tall as I could in the back seat, craning my neck, trying to catch a glimpse of them in their night world. These first sightings of nocturnal wildlife in Wales captivated me and always prevented the dark from holding much fear. Even now, if I cannot sleep, I know that the wood behind our cottage is a sort of busy bosky city at night, and I find this a very comforting thought. The call of an owl can help to banish even the most severe anxiety: the roaring, nerve-searing kind that seems to bubble up at 3 a.m.

The seas off the coast of Pembrokeshire are warmed by the Gulf Stream and as a result the biodiversity along the rocky shoreline of this part of Britain is some of the

richest in the UK. In 1991, I went on a college field trip to
Dale Fort, on St Ann's Head near Milford Haven, and was
astonished by the range of species we found: large brown
sea slugs called sea hares, little orange sponges, brittle stars
and even a worm pipefish (a cousin of seahorses with a
long thin body), lurking beneath some seaweed in a rock
pool like a living shoelace. When I was small I didn't know
much about maritime wildlife, but I knew that I could
find VERY interesting things in rock pools: things that
darted, scuttled and snailed about; that I could catch in
my net if I was careful and they'd continue to dart, scuttle
and snail about in my bucket. When I was seven, I had
been allowed to stay up to watch *Life on Earth* when it was
first shown on BBC1. I remember underwater footage of
whales, dolphins and shoals of vivid fish on coral reefs. The
miniature collections of creatures I found in Pembrokeshire
rock pools and placed, for just a short time, in my seaside
bucket were as fascinating to me as the formidable marine
creatures I had seen on the television.

One summer, it may have been 1979 or 1980, I found
a pebble with an interesting pattern on it, like several
tiny sharp volcanoes. It matched the pattern I had
seen on the boulders nearby and I liked it, so I
added it to my bucket. As I watched the shrimps
and crab I had caught scuttle about in this tiny
rock pool I had made, there was another very small
movement and the pebble seemed to shimmer a
little. I remember peering more closely, wondering
if it was an illusion caused by the movement
of the water. Then I saw the top of
one of the little volcanoes open
like a trapdoor and a tiny

fringe of pinkish tentacles emerge like a minuscule hand. It began to claw at the water above it, and each time it did so the row of tentacles disappeared inside the trapdoor. It seemed to me that something similar to the footage from *Life on Earth* had just taken place right in front of me as I squatted on the sand peering into a pint or so of seawater. The only other time I had experienced exhilaration like it was on the Twister at the fun fair. I remember thinking that what I was seeing was momentous; that tiny and wonderful things were taking place in my bucket, and that surely this was so astounding that it should be on the news. When I found out that the strange little being I had seen was a common variety of barnacle, that it had been feeding on plankton in the seawater and that there were hundreds of millions of them living on the rocky beaches of Pembrokeshire, it did nothing to dim my awe. I had witnessed a fascinating creature behaving as it would have done were I not there: it was a glimpse of nature, a scrap of wildness in a bright plastic pot. It had made me feel euphoric and I was hungry for more.

I was happiest when I was in Pembrokeshire. The range of wildlife I encountered there as a child and the rare freedom I had to explore the beaches during those annual holidays meant that I have always associated that part of the UK with contentment and intense nature-based wonder.

As August now begins, I realize that I haven't been by the sea since March, when I saw the murmuration at Minsmere.

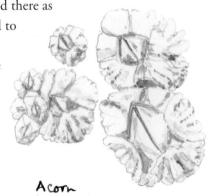

Acorn barnacle

Much as I love the Suffolk and Norfolk coastlines nearest to our cottage, for me there is a siren call from the beaches of southwest Wales: Broad Haven, Marloes, Saundersfoot, Dale, Bosherston – even their names are bewitching. I am longing to see small things dashing about in rock pools and to search for treasure along the strandline. I am longing for that sigh of mental relief that comes when I am by the sea, and in particular the coast of Pembrokeshire. Recovery from such a severe bout of depression can be a drawn-out process for mind and body. I have been tired since the spring and still don't feel fully well so I decide to head west.

I time my journey so that I arrive several hours before sunset. I am determined to visit a beach on my first evening in Pembrokeshire, and the owners of the tiny converted cow shed I am staying in point me in the direction of Wiseman's Bridge beach, a place we never visited during my childhood holidays. I set out towards the coast and within a few minutes I become aware of the distinctive raised hedgerows that line many of the roads in this part of Wales and that I remember vividly from childhood summers. At this time of year they are peppered with patches of yellow toadflax, white yarrow and mauve scabious. After I've been driving for ten minutes or so, the road begins to snake downwards towards the coast. My anticipation builds. I am about to walk on the shore. I feel childishly giddy and my mood scuds upwards like a kite. I park just a metre or two from the edge of the beach and the sea is there in front of me. The sea. I walk onto the beach and discover a sort of pavement of beautiful flattish pink and grey pebbles. They have been rounded by the waves and pressed into the sand by the passage of thousands of feet walking towards the shore. They are strewn here and there with dried seaweed, and I stand for some minutes simply looking down at them.

When I spend time on a beach, I experience a covetous feeling and want to possess the pebbles, shells, sand and small creatures that live there. Beaches cause such a dramatic and welcome shift in my brain chemistry that I long to take scraps of them home as talismans against the difficult days that are bound to come. It is a more potent version of the botanical covetousness I experienced in the village wood in November, when I felt as acquisitive towards the sloes, haws and bright leaves trimming the branches as I am towards semi-precious stones or skeins of soft yarn. This is the dopamine of beachcombing. I want to own these pebbles, line our cottage with them, arrange them into a patchwork, tailor them into a stony suit and walk around wearing them. I would look like a sort of pebbly armadillo and I think it would be the most beautiful outfit of all. I content myself with taking a photograph.

As I walk towards the sea, my feet cross from pebbles to sand, and the kite of my feelings climbs further. I see a group of pools to my right, so I make my way towards them and clamber onto the rocks to see what I can find there, as I did so many times as a child. The first small rock pool I come across is no larger than a bath mat. It's lined with seaweed and immediately I see dark red beadlet anemones attached to its gently sloping rocky walls, lying in wait for plankton to drift past their outstretched tentacles. Where the beadlets are attached above the waterline they have retracted their tentacles and look like giant fruit jelly sweets whose sugar coating has been dissolved by the sea.

I have neither a bucket nor net with me, so I squat as I did when I was small and peer into the pool. There are several shrimps chasing about; they are the colour of the sand itself and subtly speckled. When they are still they become almost invisible and I wonder at the evolution of this perfect camouflage. There is a large pebble on the floor of the pool and I shift it carefully. To my delight three crabs scuttle away, causing the shrimps to dart beneath the seaweed in alarm. The carapace of the smallest crab, the size of a peanut, is covered in a bold black-and-white pattern. It is a juvenile shore crab, the kind I used to seek out for my bucket worlds. Another of the crabs, an adult shore crab, settles on the sandy bottom of the pool and begins to make a rowing movement with its legs to submerge itself, leaving only its eyes and mouthparts protruding. I store these seemingly mundane happenings in a mental cupboard that I'll open on days when depression lurks.

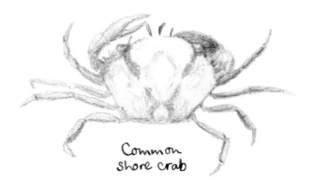

Common
shore crab

I'm keen for a paddle in the sea, so I shift position and stand up, and as I do so a pattern-seeking part of my brain lights up briefly as I glance at a crevice between two rocks. What had I seen? Some barnacles? The spiral of a whelk?

I lower myself again and look carefully. Clamped to the rock is a chiton. It is a small mollusc with eight overlapping shell plates and looks like a legless seaside woodlouse, a tiny fragment of alligator skin. The only other time I have seen a chiton is on my college field trip to Pembrokeshire, and to discover one again twenty-seven years later has a pleasing neatness to it. The earliest fossil chiton to be found is 400 million years old, so this is a modern member of a truly ancient family of animals.

I leave my sandals on a rock, roll up the legs of my jeans and paddle in the shallows for some time. Humans are drawn to water, both fresh and salt, as it would have aided our survival, but there are more benefits than simply food and hydration. The marine biologist Wallace Nichols believes that standing on the shore and looking out to sea, or watching a river as it slips by, gives our eyes and brains a break from visual stimuli. It is a holiday for the brain, a rest from the frenetic and incessant input we receive in modern life: a sort of maritime meditation. I certainly feel this as I stand there, allowing the water to wash around my feet. As the waves advance and recede, my mind drifts into a quiet stasis that feels similar to when I am crocheting or drawing. Mental din recedes and dark thoughts evaporate. I understand why the seaside was prescribed for so many ailing Victorians.

The sun is beginning to set, the light on the beach becomes golden, and as often happens when I am immersed in nature I realize I have forgotten to eat. I make my way back to the car, but peep into one last rock pool on my way up the beach. Next to the pool is a cluster of large pinkish barnacles that must have become detached. I place them in the water. I have little hope of them emerging, as the bases of several are broken and jagged where they have come away from boat or rock; two of them have holes where their trapdoors should have been and I suspect that this cluster may be dead, but I watch and wait, just in case. One of the remaining trapdoors seems to darken. It opens slightly and the barnacle begins to feed. I am reliving an encounter that I first experienced more than thirty-five years ago. As I watch this small creature have a meal I am filled with gratitude for nature's ability to mend my mind.

The next day I drive to Marloes beach. I remember these sands being punctuated with impressively huge rocks and that I saw a little dark fish lurking in a crevice in one of them, away from any rock pools, yet alive and rather wriggly when I touched it gently with some seaweed. I remember wondering at this fish. How could it survive away from water? On my college field trip I learned that it was a blenny, also known as a shanny or sea-frog. Providing their skin remains moist, these intrepid fish can escape the low oxygen levels of rock pools by wedging themselves into small rocky openings as the tide recedes, spending several hours there, safe and still until the tide rises again and they can swim away to feed. I am curious to know whether blennies still live at Marloes. In the nineties there was at least one significant oil spill from the tankers docking at Milford Haven. Perhaps this habitat no longer supports the ecological diversity that it did when I was young.

There is a mile or so to walk from the car park to Marloes beach across fields and down steep winding paths to the shore. As I walk, I notice that the landscape seems less parched here in Pembrokeshire than it does at home

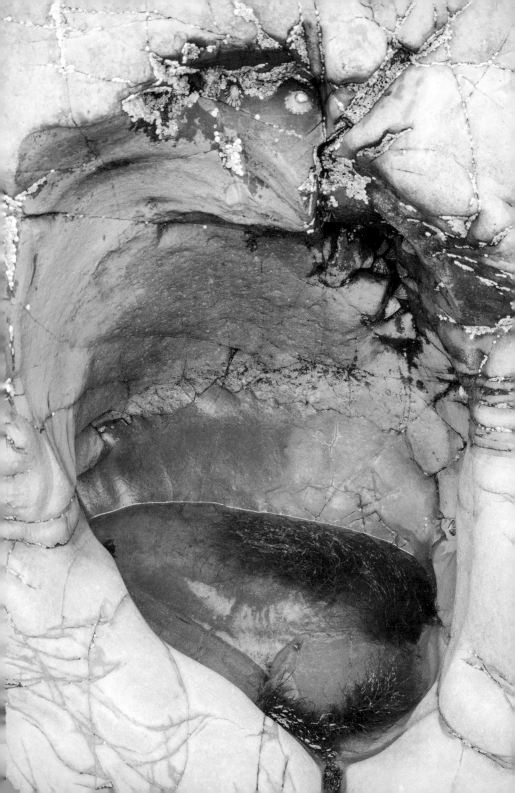

in the Fens. It is lush and verdant, as though we had not had two months of scorching temperatures. Perhaps the nearby Preseli Hills have triggered more rainfall here than in Eastern England. It is a relief to my senses to see so many shades of green after the desiccated grasses of Cambridgeshire. As I approach the beach I turn a corner in the path and my eyes are met with a view that I haven't seen in over three decades. I'm overwhelmed by memory and emotion, the fragrant smell of dry coastal grassland, the subtle pink of thrift flowers on a cliff, the movement of a tiny fish, seawater trapped in rocks pitted and hollowed out by waves, the tang of drying seaweed, a tiny cushion star held reverently in my palm as though it were an emerald. Seeking out repetition of the piercing joy of my first encounters with nature, experienced here at Marloes and in my grandad's garden, has helped me to keep on living. This place holds enormous meaning for me.

The rocks at Marloes are like a geological hallucination. The strata have been shifted through 90° by the earth's heave, and they undulate wildly. Enormous sea-worn chunks of this layered stone erupt from the sand like the bodies of prehistoric reptiles. The rocks are encrusted with a chain mail of barnacles, and the pools that form in and around them are teeming with life. Some are several metres tall, all are a deep red with stripes of mustard and grey and are worn smooth by millennia of waves and scouring sands. There are crevices along them where some of the upended strata have been eroded more quickly. Here, long shallow pools form, full of candy-striped winkles, beadlet anemones, an intricate barnacle crust and

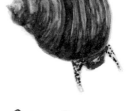

Common
periwinkle

< Rock pool at Marloes beach, Pembrokeshire

complex interconnected food webs of algae, plankton, crustaceans and fish. The rocks rise sharply from the sand, causing eddies at their bases, resulting in deep rock pools that can hold much more oxygen while the tide is out than a shallow pool a few centimetres deep.

I am examining a deep fissure in one of the rocks as I walk around it and inadvertently step into one of these pools. The sand falls away steeply at its edge and I nearly stumble. As I steady myself I peer into it. Immediately adjacent to the rock the water is deep enough to have a blue tinge, and the range of life here is remarkable. I can see the darting movements of fish around five or six inches long, at least three varieties of seaweed, small shoals of shrimps in the shallows, and the pool's rocky edge is studded with innumerable whelks and winkles. Suddenly a tiny plaice, the size of a fifty pence piece, swims out across the pool just beneath the surface. Like the shrimps in these rock pools, it is the exact colour of sand, with subtle pale spots on its skin. A muscular sine wave crosses and re-crosses its body, propelling it gracefully through the water. I have never seen a flatfish in a rock pool before and I gasp with excitement. It glides towards the edge of the pool and settles on the sand, shivering its body slightly to cause a cloud of grains to rise around it and fall onto its back. It is instantly invisible.

I have looked into several crevices in the rocks, hoping to see a blenny, but have spotted nothing but anemones and limpets

Bladderwrack

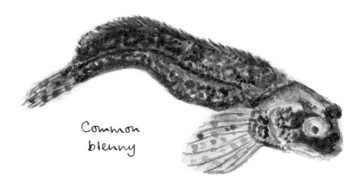

Common
blenny

lurking there. I am on the verge of giving up and returning to the car. As I start to make my way back to the path down to the beach, I pass one of the largest rocks. There is a deep but very narrow gorge in it where a softer geological layer has been worn away by endless tides. I peep in. A small dark frog-like face peers balefully back at me. A blenny. I pick up a piece of seaweed as I did when I was small and move it gently towards the fish. To my astonishment it bites violently at the frond of weed, making a loud snapping sound with its jaws, which are designed to crunch barnacles off rocks. I recoil, thrilled by this little creature's audacity. My encounter with both the feeding barnacle and this little fish hiding in a hole in a rock have echoed my childhood experiences in Pembrokeshire and reassured me that the habitats on these shores are as rich with wildlife as they were in the late 1970s. My trip to the beaches of West Wales has been curative. It has left me feeling well for the first time since last autumn.

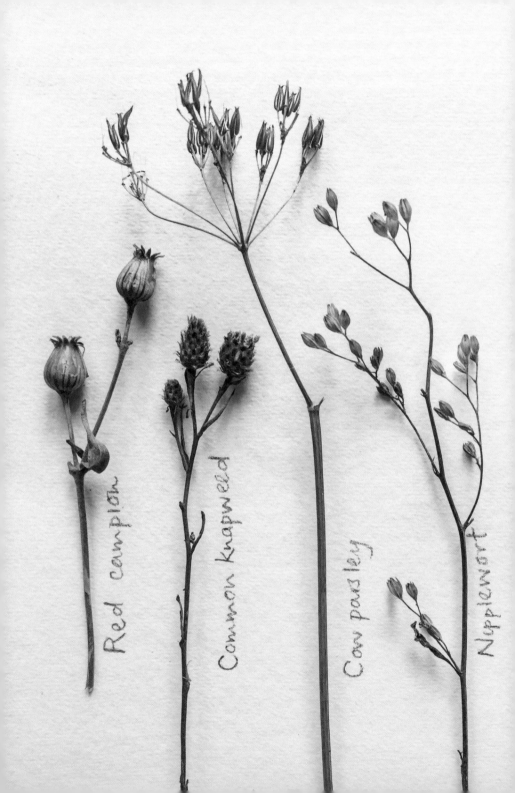

Red campion

Common knapweed

Cow parsley

Nipplewort

September

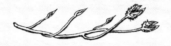

Blackberries ripen.
Swallows prepare to leave.

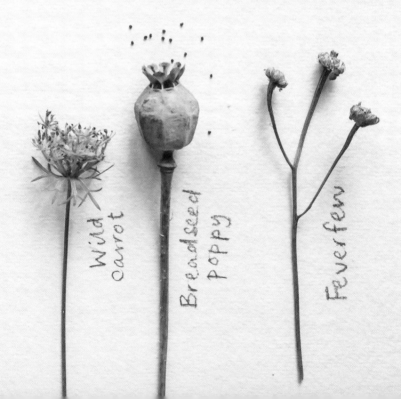

Wild carrot

Breadseed poppy

Feverfew

The heatwave is over. It was broken by storms and torrential rain in late August, and the countryside has been gently returning to green. Showers have revived the cutting flowers I sowed in April and May, and they have begun to bloom again. I'm sitting on a newly built step in our garden and am surrounded by bright spots of colour: oranges and yellows from marigolds, pinks from cosmos, blues from borage and cornflowers, and the ethereal yellow umbels of fennel. The searing temperatures of June, July and August have been replaced by a gentle warmth, and the light has begun to soften and become golden as we move towards autumn. Over the last months, while my recovery has continued and I've been writing this book, I have come into the garden for a few minutes most days.

It is human-made, this place. We have transformed a long, narrow, steeply sloping strip of land into four levels of brick, wood, turf and soil. Yet there is wildness here. A family of bank voles has built a network of burrows next to the small shed that houses the boiler. The adult voles go out to forage each day for themselves and for their young I hope they are stowing below the surface of my flowerbeds. A week or two ago I looked out of the living room window to see one of them shinning up one of our tomato plants, as though it were a tree, to pilfer the ripe fruit. My youngest daughter had been wondering why the choicest tomatoes kept disappearing. A juvenile toad regularly appears at the back door, where there is a damp patch of ground, and several mason bees have made their nests in the drilled logs we added to the wall that was built a few months ago. Small bird stories unfold in the garden each day: the rage of the resident male blackbird towards all corvids and starlings, the affable flocks of goldfinches and long-tailed tits that visit the bird feeders, the dunnock that creeps beneath the plants, and the wren that lurks and feeds among the ivy that forms our boundary with next door. Innumerable bees, butterflies, hoverflies, ladybirds and less showy insects live in and visit these few tens of square metres of garden.

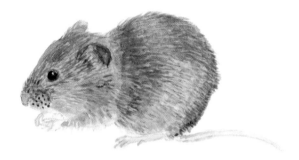

Bank vole

I let all seedlings that germinate in our patch have their chance, then I edit later. Many may think the garden is messy in places, but I have gained numerous free plants this way. Seeds travel here on the wind, in the digestive tracts of birds and small mammals, and they stow away in plant pots from car boot sales and roadside honesty stalls. My method is to stop weeding for weeks and sometimes months on end, and then remove some of the nettles, most of the thistles and as much bindweed and ground elder as I can manage. Nature seems to relish my approach. I have unwittingly provided habitats for a wide range of species by letting a botanical medley develop.

Watching the behaviour and interactions of the inhabitants of our garden has been a source of solace for me in recent months. I am living proof of the research undertaken by the University of Exeter, showing that

seeing plants, trees, and watching wildlife, can help to
lift depression. There is no doubt that spending time in a
wild landscape benefits the mind, but simply looking at
wild happenings through your kitchen window will help if
depression has you in its steely grip.

As I sit with a cup of tea, I can hear the chatter of
swallows as they embroider the sky with their flight
lines high above my head. There is a comforting familiar
whistling babble from goldfinches in the crab-apple tree
and a soporific cooing from a collared dove in the hedge.
Then a thin, sharp, undulating call pierces the air in the
garden. It sounds like a wren, yet it is far quieter, faltering.
I hold my breath as I listen. The wren's characteristic trill
is there among the cacophony of notes, then the song
trails off. I am puzzled. A wren's song in the breeding
season is strident, confident and surprisingly loud given

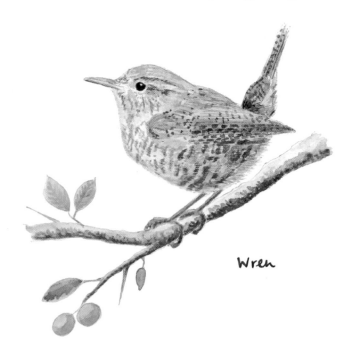

Wren

the bird's size. Most birds cease their songs in July
once their broods have fledged. Earlier in the year they
would have been expending energy in proclaiming their
territories or advertising to mates, but in late summer
these are not priorities. Instead, they moult their feathers
and hide in foliage and hedges. Gardens and countryside
can seem very quiet in late summer, as many birds are
silent and some will not begin to sing again until the
following February or March, when the breeding season
begins. What I'm hearing now is what's called a sub-song,
sometimes believed to be a kind of 'practice' song. It
could even be one of this year's juveniles, testing out his
tweeting prowess. This sound is all the more bewitching
for its imperfection, the near silence of the surrounding
countryside, and the thought that this could be one of the
first times this bird has ever uttered a note.

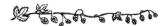

Until I began to discover bee orchids in our village
wood, my knowledge of this group of plants was scant.
These small exotic-seeming flowers growing so close to
our cottage inspired me to find out more about what
is perhaps the most captivating family of wildflowers
growing in the UK. I learned that there were tall lizard
orchids growing on the edge of Newmarket racecourse,
speckled with patterns like reptile skin and smelling
rather rankly of goats. I visited the early purple orchids
that open in April and grow in the glades of Bradfield
Woods. I read about the common spotted-orchid and
how it can confound botanists by crossing with the marsh
orchid, and I gazed at pictures of the ethereal green

twayblades that lurk in ancient woodlands. I had always assumed that the flowering season of British orchids was confined to the middle of the year; that once the last of the summer-flowering species faded on the Hebrides, orchids would not appear in the botanical calendar again until the early purples opened the following spring. This year I have learned that there is a summer straggler, an orchid species that begins to bloom in late August.

Like many of the species I saw at Rose End Meadows in June, autumn lady's-tresses grows in calcareous grassland habitats that have not been treated with fertilizers. It needs the biodiversity of microflora and fungi that comes from untouched soil in order to flourish. As with several of the species or habitats I have sought this year, I learned of its existence from Twitter and set about finding the flowering site nearest our cottage. My friend Isabella and I decide to head to a small nature reserve in Bedfordshire called Knocking Hoe.

There are no signs to direct us to the reserve. Finding it becomes a test of our ability to stitch together several sets of vague directions, fragments of information from Google maps and accounts from locals of a 'bun-shaped hill'. We start down a track marked 'private road', and after walking half a mile or so we reach a farm and are informed that we're trespassing. I confess I become secretly gleeful at this point. We're being told off for orchid hunting. It seems like something that might have happened in the nineteenth century. I apologize to the farmer, assure him that we wish no harm to his land, and declare that we will find another way back from the reserve.

We emerge from behind a barn and there in front of us ... is a bun-shaped hill. There are still no signs, but we feel this must be the place, so we press on and head towards a gate at the base of the hill. In the field beyond are cows. Isabella is not keen on ruminants, especially when they gallop across fields and loom behind stiles, so we find a path that arcs widely to our right and follows a ridge of land that meets the crest of the hill. Along the edge of the path there are still points of colour from late summer wildflowers: devil's bit scabious, clustered bellflower, agrimony and the tiny white lobelia-like flowers of eyebright. As we climb the ridge, beautiful views open up across the county. The sky has a pearly opalescence in places but most of it is a steely grey. I worry it might rain.

We reach the summit and there is a sign confirming we are at Knocking Hoe. We pass through the gate and follow a path across the hill. The land falls away steeply to our left. Optimistically, I thought the autumn lady's-tresses would be easy to find and might be visible among the grasses as soon as we entered the reserve. We continue walking and I leave the path several times to search for this elusive flower, but find only wild roses with an occasional robin's pincushion, harebells and patches of Breckland thyme. As lovely as these plants are, we're beginning to feel frustrated at the dearth of orchids, the sky is darkening and we feel the first raindrops. I'm concerned that we're on a floral wild goose chase, are stuck at the top of a hill with only one coat in dingy weather and are now two miles from where we parked. We reach an electric fence with a sort of handmade rustic stile set in it. In the steeply sloping field beyond, several tens of small red flags have been pushed into the ground. I wonder if these mark the positions of orchids and we venture into the field to find out.

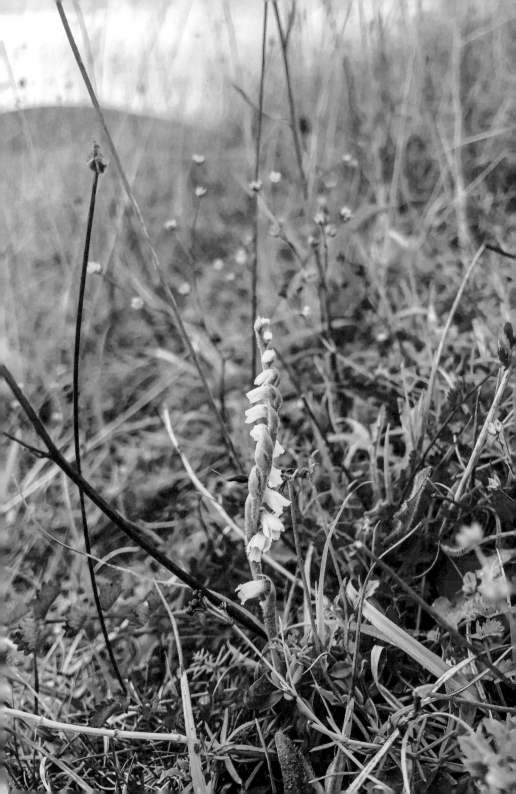

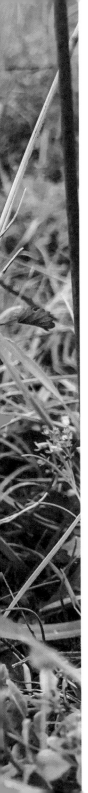

When autumn lady's-tresses first appeared on my Twitter feed there was no way of telling its size, and I assumed it was as tall and showy as a bee orchid. I approach the nearest red flag carefully, as the incline in this field means that I struggle to keep a foothold as I climb down, even in sturdy boots. My eyes detect a pattern of pale dots very close to the ground and next to the flag. I drop down to examine the pattern more closely and find an exquisite string of very tiny white orchid flowers just 5 mm in diameter spiralling round a stem that is the pale bluish grey of an olive leaf. The foliage is covered in a down of very fine hairs that make it look as though it is covered in frost. This specimen of autumn lady's-tresses is no more than 8 cm high. I had no idea orchids could be this small. This species is relatively rare in the UK as it requires untreated calcareous grassland in which to grow, and such sites are now scarce. I crouch even closer to the ground to take a picture of this specimen and its neighbour a few metres away, and can just about detect the coconut scent it produces. I turn to talk to Isabella further up the slope and see another floral helix, even smaller than the first, that has not been marked with a flag. I've discovered an unseen orchid on this hill.

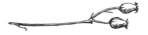

I end my year the way I began it, walking up to the wood behind our cottage with Annie. The spindle leaves are beginning to show hems of pink, the sloes are coated in bloom that seems to enhance

‹ Autumn lady's-tresses at Knocking Hoe nature reserve

their blueness, and the scabious seed heads are drying in the warmth of the early autumn sun. This place is part of me. It is fundamental to my connection with nature and has been crucial to my recovery since March. The five-minute walk from our house to this patch of trees is one I take when the world seems disjointed and broken and my dark thoughts implacable. When I catch sight of the common plants that grow in this stretch of land – clover, black medick, wild rose, knapweed, cow parsley, blackthorn – the patterns made by their leaves, the subtle splashes of colour from their flowers and the multitude of greens, it has a unique capacity to quieten my thoughts. Walking the paths here is like a mantra for my mind made of a pattern of steps among a pattern of trees: it is soothingly repetitive and familiar, a sort of ambulatory sylvan yoga. It is as consoling as the small ritual of making tea or the conjuring of loops of yarn into a mitten, yet each time it is different. Today, a pair of small heath butterflies are twirling in a late mating dance above some ragwort, and I spy an adult muntjac again in the patch of fenced-off trees where the large snowdrops flowered in February.

The plants that grow in these few hectares of native trees are beginning to show signs of autumn, yet summer is still here in the late flowers of the hedge-parsley, the delicate pink-mauve of the blue fleabane and the yellow of hawkbits. This is a cusp between two seasons and the wood is beautiful. Annie and I begin to make our way home. I know colder days are approaching, and as ever I am daunted by the onset of winter, but being in nature has healed my broken mind this year. On its darkest day in

March it was the sight of some saplings and their soothing
greenness in the central reservation of a dual carriageway
that altered the tone of my thoughts and ushered me away
from the brink of suicide. The last twelve months have
been so difficult that it felt unreal, horrifying; I have felt
dissociated from much of it, but each time I have faltered,
the sight of a bird or a brief walk among trees has shifted
my mental gears away from the worst manifestations
of depression. This knowledge gives me enormous
reassurance. Wild places are an essential medicine for me, a
sort of safety net.

This year of using nature as a remedy has convinced me
that humans may need to be in natural landscapes regularly
in order to be fully well. There is an ancient and potent
connection between us and the land: we evolved to live in
wild places. Perhaps it is the displacement from nature in
modern life that is causing so many of us to struggle with
our mental health.

The incidence of mental illness is increasing in the
world's population. It is unclear exactly why this is
occurring and theories abound: we are more isolated from
community structures, the digital age has cultivated new
social pressures and demands on our time, modern diets
have altered our brain chemistry, life is more stressful
than it was for previous generations. But what is clear to
me and the many who have conducted research in the
area, is that whatever other factors have played their part,
our disconnection from nature holds a critical
role in this story. The author Richard Louv has
proposed that human health, especially that of
children, is suffering because we spend less time
outdoors. He called this Nature Deficit Disorder.

Our hunter-gatherer ancestors would have spent a large proportion of their days on the shore or among trees, and once the earliest farmers began to settle and cultivate the land, the lives of humans continued to be intimately entwined with many elements of their environment: bodies of water, forests, plants, and the animals that lived in these habitats. Humans evolved to live this way. To expect that we would have no ill effects from being transplanted into new environments and ways of life so devoid of time spent in nature is surely unreasonable.

There is an interconnected array of physiological and neurological changes that take place within us when we move from our homes, offices or an urban environment into a place with trees, verdure and wildlife. The science is still progressing but several strands of research have shown that we could begin to harness the beneficial effects of wild places to help allay mental illness. I'm fully aware that it may not have the transformative impact for everyone that it has for me, but my hope is that taking walks in nature will become a much more widespread response to a depression diagnosis; that it will stop being regarded as something unusual, with a hint of eccentricity, and that instead this knowledge, these clues at the fundamental need for humans to be outdoors, will begin to be used as an effective treatment for mental illness alongside standard medical and psychotherapeutic approaches.

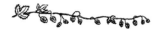

The blackberries are beginning to ripen in the wood, and I stop to pick and eat some, allowing the September sun to warm my back. Annie prods her nose into the undergrowth beneath a guelder-rose tree festooned with clusters of beautiful translucent red berries. Her snout suddenly points upwards in high alert as a squirrel becomes aware of her and scampers up the trunk in alarm. They stare at each other, squirrel in the tree, Annie on the ground, in a sort of mammalian stand-off for several seconds before the squirrel takes a leap into a cherry tree on the other side of the path and disappears out of sight. A speckled wood butterfly lands on a blackberry leaf to bask in the sun and a southern hawker flits along the path ahead of me.

Annie and I amble round the last corner of the path leading back to our house. I hear a chattering to my right and look over a hedge to see swallows gathering on parallel telephone wires, like notes on a stave. They are readying themselves for the journey ahead. In a very few weeks they will leave for another year.

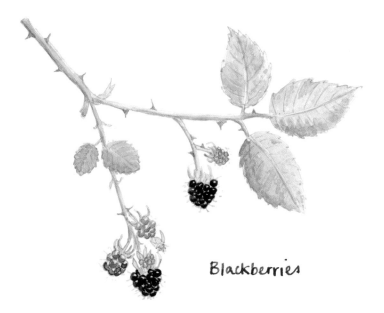

Blackberries

Bibliography

Shepherd, Nan, *The Living Mountain* (Aberdeen, 1977).

Shinrin-yoku / Forest bathing

Hansen, M. M., Jones, R. and Tocchini, K., 'Shinrin-Yoku (Forest Bathing) and Nature Therapy: A State-of-the-Art review', *International Journal of Environmental Research and Public Health*, August 2017, 14(8): 851.

The effects of phytoncides on the immune system

Li Q., Kobayashi M., Wakayama Y., Inagaki, H., Katsumata M., Hirata Y., Shimizu T., Kawada T., Park B. J., Ohira T., Kagawa T. and Miyazaki Y., 'Effect of phytoncide from trees on human natural killer cell function', *International Journal of Immunopathology and Pharmacology*, October–December 2009, 22(4): 951–9.

The benefits to humans of interactions with natural landscapes

Beyer, K. M., Kaltenback, A., Szabo, A., Bogar, S., Nieto, F. J. and Malecki, K. M., 'Exposure to neighborhood green space and mental health: evidence from the survey of the health of Wisconsin', *International Journal of Environmental Research into Public Health*, March 2014, 11(3): 3453–72.

Cox, D. T. C., Shanahan, D. F., Hudson, H. L., Plummer, K. E., Siriwardena, G. M., Fuller, R. A., Anderson, K., Hancock, S. and Gaston, K. J., 'Doses of Neighborhood Nature: The Benefits for Mental Health of Living with Nature', *BioScience*, vol 67, issue 2, February 2017, pp. 147–155.

Johnston, Ian, 'Human brain hard-wired for rural tranquility', *Independent*, 10 December 2013.

Keniger, L. E., Gaston, K. J., Irvine, K. N. and Fuller, R. A., 'What are the Benefits of Interacting with Nature?', *International Journal of Environmental Research into Public Health*, March 2013, 10(3): 913–935.

Velarde, M. D., Fry, G. and Tveit, M., 'Health effects of viewing landscapes: Landscape types in environmental psychology', *Urban Forestry and Urban Greening*, vol 6, issue 4, November 2007, pp. 199–212.

Role of the serotoninergic system on mood and mood disorders

Albert, P. R. and Benkelfat, C., 'The neurobiology of depression – revisiting the serotonin hypothesis. II. Genetic, epigenetic and clinical studies', *Philosophical Transactions of the Royal Society B: Biological Sciences*, April 2013, 368(1615): 20120535.

Blier, P. and El Mansari, M., 'Serotonin and beyond: therapeutics for major depression', *Philosophical Transactions of the Royal Society B: Biological Sciences*, February 2013, 368(1615): 20120536.

Sansone, R. A. and Sansone, L. A., 'Sunshine, Serotonin and Skin: A Partial Explanation for Seasonal Patterns in Psychopathology?', *Innovations in Clinical Neuroscience*, July–August 2013, 10(7–8): 20–24.

Young, S. N., 'The effect of raising and lowering tryptophan levels on human mood and social behaviour', *Philosophical Transactions of the Royal Society B: Biological Sciences*, February 2013, 368(1615): 20110375.

Link between gut flora and serotonin

Jenkins, T. A., Nguyen, J. C. D., Polglaze, K. E. and Bertrand, P. P., 'Influence of Tryptophan and Serotonin on Mood and Cognition with a Possible Role of the Gut-Brain Axis', *Nutrients*, January 2016, 8(1): 56.

Biochemical changes in the suicidal brain

Wenner, Melinda, 'The Origins of Suicidal Brains', *Scientific American*, 1 February 2009.

Harvest high and dopamine release on exploring / exploiting local resources

Barack, D. L. and Platt, M. L., 'Engaging and Exploring: Cortical Circuits for Adaptive Foraging Decisions', *Impulsivity*, vol 64, 2017, pp. 163–199.

Francis, Robyn, 'Why Gardening Makes You Happy and Cures Depression', Permaculture College Australia, permaculture.com.au.

McClure, S. M., Gilzenrat, M. S. and Cohen, J. D., 'An exploration-exploitation model based on norepinepherine and dopamine activity', *Advances in Neural Information Processing Systems*, 2005.

Repetitive movements of hand and eye and their effects on serotonin

Jacobs, B. L., 'Serotonin, Motor Activity and Depression-Related Disorders', *American Scientist*, vol 82, no 5, September–October 1994, pp. 456–463.

Acknowledgements

Thank you to Andy, Evie and Rose, who have been immensely patient and supportive while I've made this book.

Charlotte Newland, Rachael Maslen, Helen Ayres, Sarah Phelps, Isabella Streffen, Jane Pink, Josie George and Melissa Harrison have cheered me on and encouraged me throughout this process. Their kindness has been invaluable.

Boundless thanks to my agent, Juliet Pickering, who continues to have faith in my writing and ideas and to my editor, Fiona Slater, whose tireless guidance has made this book readable. Neither *The Wild Remedy* nor *Making Winter* would look so beautiful without the humbling and wizard-like design skills and patience of Claire Cater.

Without the supportive words and encouragement of friends I've met on Twitter and Instagram, it's doubtful whether this book would exist. Thank you.

A final thank you to Annie, my slightly niffy, hairy pal, who is always keen to walk with me.

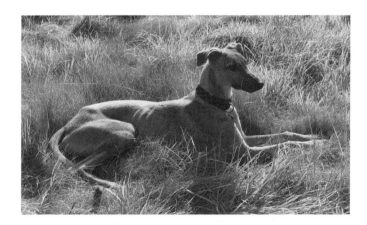